STAFF
RAMPTON

D1759710

The Neuroscience of Psychological Therapies

The Neuroscience of Psychological Therapies summarizes knowledge of brain function and brain behavior relationships within the context of psychotherapy implementation. It describes how specific locations in the brain carry out specific activities, how the different activities are combined to yield normal and pathological behavior, and how knowledge of brain activities can guide psychological assessment and intervention. Specific topics include the influence of neural networks on discovery and change, the therapist's neuroscience, communicating with patients using the brain as reference, and using neuroscience concepts to compare and integrate traditional schools of psychotherapy. Applying a neuroscience framework to conceptualization and treatment of depression is offered as an example, and specific issues associated with trauma and false memories are discussed. The book is aimed at anyone who is working within a psychotherapy framework and wishes to discover more about brain function and brain/behavior relationships.

Rowland W. Folensbee is a Clinical Associate Professor in the Menninger Department of Psychiatry and Behavioral Sciences at Baylor College of Medicine, Houston, Texas. He maintains a private practice in psychology and consults in schools. He received his doctorate in psychology from The Pennsylvania State University. His training included behavioral, cognitive behavioral, and psychodynamic approaches. His passion for the past 20 years has been the integration of neuropsychology and neuroscience into clinical assessment and intervention. One of his primary goals has been to translate this integration into language that can be understood and used by lay persons and clinicians who are not immersed in the complex world of the brain. The present book is the product of his passion.

WITHDRAWN
FROM
DMH STAFF LIBRARY

LIBRARY RAMPTON HOSPITAL

R77763

The Neuroscience of Psychological Therapies

Rowland W. Folensbee

Menninger Department of Psychiatry
and Behavioral Sciences
Baylor College of Medicine

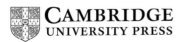

CAMBRIDGE UNIVERSITY PRESS
Cambridge, New York, Melbourne, Madrid, Cape Town, Singapore, São Paulo

Cambridge University Press
The Edinburgh Building, Cambridge CB2 8RU, UK

Published in the United States of America by Cambridge University Press, New York

www.cambridge.org
Information on this title: www.cambridge.org/9780521863179

© R. W. Folensbee 2007

This publication is in copyright. Subject to statutory exception
and to the provisions of relevant collective licensing agreements,
no reproduction of any part may take place without
the written permission of Cambridge University Press.

First published 2007

Printed in the United Kingdom at the University Press, Cambridge

A catalog record for this publication is available from the British Library

Library of Congress Cataloging in Publication data

Folensbee, Rowland W.
The neuroscience of psychological therapies / Rowland W. Folensbee.
  p. ; cm.
Includes bibliographical references.
ISBN-13: 978-0-521-86317-9 (hardback)
ISBN-10: 0-521-86317-1 (hardback)
ISBN-13: 978-0-521-68188-9 (pbk.)
ISBN-10: (invalid) 0-521-68188-2 (pbk.)
1. Neuropsychology. 2. Psychotheraphy. 3. Neurosciences. I. Title.
[DNLM: 1. Neuropsychology—methods. 2. Brain—physiology. 3. Nerve Net—physiology.
4. Psychotheraphy—methods. WL 103.5 F663a 2006]

QP360.F65 2007
612.8–dc22

2006102402

ISBN-13 978-0-521-86317-9   hardback
ISBN-13 978-0-521-68188-9   paperback

Cambridge University Press has no responsibility for the persistence or accuracy of URLs
for external or third-party internet websites referred to in this publication, and does not
guarantee that any content on such websites is, or will remain, accurate or appropriate.

Every effort has been made in preparing this book to provide accurate and up-to-date
information that is in accord with accepted standards and practice at the time of publication.
Nevertheless, the authors, editors and publishers can make no warranties that the information
contained herein is totally free from error, not least because clinical standards are constantly
changing through research and regulation. The authors, editors and publishers therefore
disclaim all liability for direct or consequential damages resulting from the use of material
contained in this book. Readers are strongly advised to pay careful attention to information
provided by the manufacturer of any drugs or equipment that they plan to use.

To my wife, Flossy,

to my children, Tre, Tyler, Matt, and Meredith,

to my father, Rowland,

and in memory of my mother, Adelaide

Contents

Acknowledgements

This book is the culmination of 20 years of somewhat meandering exploration of connections between the brain and behavior. During those years my understanding of the brain has been cobbled onto and worked into my ongoing clinical practice. The path toward the future of this enterprise was often poorly defined, although it rested firmly on an intuition that understanding connections between the brain and experiences of psychotherapy could guide clinical activity. I want to acknowledge those who contributed to this exploration, often in ways not directly tied to neuroscience.

The graduate training program in clinical psychology at The Pennsylvania State University offered a milieu in which students were encouraged to find their unique paths into the field, and this approach set the stage for my subsequent exploration of neuroscience and psychotherapy. Tom Borkovec, Steve Danish, and Juris Draguns were Penn State mentors who supported my personal explorations, offering models of respectful competence within individual fields of clinical study while simultaneously encouraging learning outside their own approaches to therapy. Beyond the realm of clinical application, Paul Cornwell demonstrated that exuberance and exploration of the brain belonged together.

I was in the audience during two presentations that particularly stimulated the subsequent development of my ideas related to clinical application of neuroscience. Gordon Bower offered the concept of neural networks during a visit to Penn State in the early 1980s. He was careful not to describe networks as biological fact, but the concept took root in my initial conceptualizations of how the brain supports experience. Daniel Siegel's presentation to the American Association of Directors of Psychiatric Residency Training in 1996 offered a description of how memory processes, trauma, and psychotherapy could interact. His ideas added to mine and simultaneously encouraged my own continuing exploration along similar paths.

More recently, the positive responses and suggestions of two clinical researcher/practitioners guided me to specific sources of information and, more importantly, offered the encouragement I needed to pursue the publication of this book. Glen Gabbard's ideas regarding the neuroscience basis for psychodynamic processes combined with his suggestions for reading and his positive response to my ideas helped me reach the point of submitting a proposal for publication. Lauren Marengel's positive responses during discussions of my ideas helped maintain my motivation, and her guidance toward specific resources regarding depression helped me elaborate ideas found in the chapter on applying neuroscience to the treatment of depression.

Trainees and fellow clinicians offered support, assistance, and, at times, a generous portion of doubt regarding the relevance of neuroscience for psychological therapies. Both the support and the questioning helped me shape my ideas into a form that I hope is relevant to the typical practicing clinician and the traditional trainee. Gordon Bush worked to keep me from slipping too far from the facts and into the art of clinical intervention. Hope Caperton-Brown, Brad Frank, and Traci Gibert each took time to review the manuscript through the eyes of clinician or trainee less familiar with, and sometimes even skeptical of, the idea that neuroscience can be immediately relevant to treatment. Their feedback shaped the final form this book has assumed.

Martin Griffiths, my editor with Cambridge University Press, emerged as an unexpected staunch advocate in the process of having my proposal accepted for publication. His support from the research side of the chasm between clinicians and researchers has encouraged within me the idea that bridges across this chasm can be built. It is thanks to him that I have begun to imagine that a description of the connections between the brain and clinical work may help researchers as well as clinicians.

Finally, without the support of my wife, Flossy, and my four children, Tre, Tyler, Matt, and Meredith, this book would never have emerged. The time taken to write this book has often been wrenched from time that could have been spent with the family. Their indulgence ("It's okay. Dad is just talking about the brain again.") of my obsession with the brain has been immeasurably helpful. Beyond the support she has given as my wife, Flossy has offered further support in her role as Director of Child Psychiatry Training at Baylor College of Medicine. Her positive responses to my presentation of these ideas at national training forums and to presentations offered to the psychiatry and psychology trainees at Baylor have provided invaluable encouragement while also providing settings in which my ideas could develop to the point they have reached today.

Introduction

Knowledge of brain structure and function has developed rapidly in recent decades; accompanying this increase in knowledge has been the rapid development of our understanding of how brain function relates to human behavior. The roles of specific areas of the brain in specific types of cognitive and emotional processes have been delineated and the complex patterns of interaction between specific areas of the nervous system required for thought and behavior have been increasingly well identified. Processes at the molecular and cellular levels and their relationships to memory, cognition, and affect have been described with increasing clarity. The biological underpinnings of specific psychiatric and neurological disorders have been outlined, and these findings have directly led to improvements in medical, psychological, and behavioral interventions for the various disorders.

The host of advances in the understanding of connections between the brain and behavior can support psychotherapeutic conceptualization and intervention (e.g. Cozolino, 2002; Pliszka, 2003). However, it is the author's experience that the vastness of the relevant literature combined with the complexity of the relationships between brain function and behavior, affect, and cognition serve to preclude the use of such understanding by many practicing clinicians. The terms alone are frightening: dorsolateral prefrontal cortex, superior temporal gyrus, ventricular epithelium. The steps and interactions in the brain comprising so basic a task as focusing attention (Posner & Raichle, 1994) can leave a clinician feeling hopeless in regard to ever understanding enough about the brain to apply such information to clinical intervention. During discussions with fellow clinicians, a moment of early interest seen in a colleague's eye quickly glazes over, turning into blank dullness reflecting a brain that has escaped from a task that seems impossible and therefore irrelevant.

This book has emerged from the author's experiences as a clinician struggling to grasp the implications of "the brain" for psychotherapy intervention. Early in the struggle, jumping from a morning of reading anatomy and physiology into an afternoon of psychotherapy sessions was like leaping from one planet to another. The two worlds seemed to have no connection at all, and the endeavor was fueled primarily by the author's sense of intrigue with the assumption that all of those therapy events must eventually rest on the activity of a collection of bundles and strands in a person's head. As time passed, concepts related to brain function began to intrude here and there into the author's therapy at points where sessions had previously been guided by an eclectic integration of traditional theories including psychodynamic psychotherapy and cognitive behavioral therapy. Discussing the brain helped to explain free association in terms of connections between neural networks. "Thought substitution" seemed to make more sense and to be more easily applied when described in relation to switching from one neural network to another. These brain "intrusions" into the author's psychotherapy have finally increased to the point that concepts of neuroscience are woven into clinical reflections and interventions at practically every turn, informing insights and intuitions as well as offering avenues for communication not previously available. Neuroscience has become one of the primary tools in the author's clinical armamentarium.

When this author first began reflecting on the possibility of viewing psychotherapy through the lenses of neuroscience, there was a fear that increasing consideration of brain function would lead to coldness and estrangement in the psychotherapy process. It has been surprising that the opposite has been the case. For example, empathy with a client being overwhelmed by flashbacks of previous trauma has seemed stronger when this author has reflected on the implications of research indicating that visual cortex used to encode current information is also required for recall of memories of previously established visual images; while being used during visual memory of a traumatic event, visual cortex is unlikely to be available for processing of current experience. How frightening it must be not to be able to see the therapist even though the client can hear the therapist's voice "in the distance" during a flashback. Clients have seemed remarkably reassured when their inability to see the therapist is explained in terms of possible brain mechanisms for such an experience; the apparently "crazy" experience of not being able to see someone sitting in front of them now makes sense. Considering neuroscience has led not to estrangement but to warm connection, a deeper sense of understanding, and improved ability to offer support during difficult times.

The purpose of this book is to provide a useful set of neuroscience concepts with a minimum of technical labels and without the detail that would be needed in order to make explanations anatomically or physiologically correct. The state of neuroscience research offers empirical support only for limited and specific aspects of intervention in psychotherapy;

the concepts to be presented are not "evidence-based psychotherapy". There is no chapter on "brain-based psychotherapy" in the most recent *Bergin and Garfield's Handbook of Psychotherapy and Behavior Change* (Lambert, 2004), and the current monograph does not provide information based on controlled clinical trials of therapy intervention. However, even in their present nascent state, current brain–behavior concepts can offer psychotherapists practical guidance that can be combined with previous training in traditional models of psychotherapy to yield new insights that have the potential to result in improved intervention.

This book will describe several ways of viewing connections between brain function and behavior, and will then outline how these various ways of viewing connections can contribute to psychotherapy intervention. A broad, neuropsychologically based conceptualization of the way the brain processes information will be outlined. The concept of neural networks related to individual experiences will be delineated. Memory, affect, and anxiety will be described with specific focus on ties between brain function and human experience in each area. Relevant concepts of brain development will be outlined. Once these basic areas have been outlined, connections between these concepts and human experience and behavior will be presented. Finally, implications for psychotherapeutic intervention will be discussed.

It is extremely difficult for people who are unfamiliar with the structure and function of the brain to maintain a clear picture of how the brain and its various processing systems interact. Figure 1.1 presents a simplistic diagram of the brain with labels of function applied to areas related to various types of processing. It identifies areas related to basic cognitive processes, including attention, primary sensory processing, association areas where information is integrated, and motor areas that guide many sorts of behavioral output. Figure 1.1 also identifies processes related to personal and emotional processing, including arousal centers in the brainstem, emotion and anxiety centers in the middle part of the brain, areas of the brain that are related to attachment, and areas in the frontal lobes related to decision making and executive functioning. The purpose of this diagram is not to clearly delineate all of the areas of the brain that contribute to each function. Rather, the figure identifies the basic processes to be developed in this book, and identifies a central area related to each of these functions. If the reader completed a test on brain function using this figure as the guide, failure would be the likely result since most of the processes labeled rely on interactions between multiple areas of the brain in order to carry out the specific function. Readers will not want their personal neurosurgeons to use this figure to guide a laser or a scalpel. The purpose of this visual labeling is to help the reader clearly conceptualize the nature of the division of activity among processes, and to develop a concrete

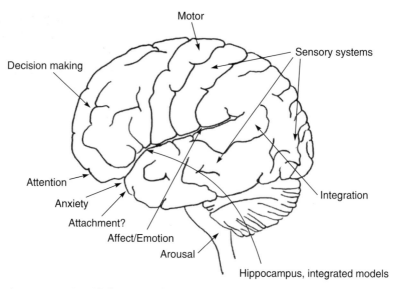

Figure 1.1 Brain with functions schematically represented.

conceptualization of how these areas and functions may relate to each other. It will be useful to return frequently to this diagram in order to maintain orientation to the basic structures and functions of the brain.

This book cannot substitute for in-depth training in the various areas that will be touched by the necessarily cursory outline to be offered. Rather, the goal of this book is to offer a framework that psychotherapists can use as they begin to apply concepts of brain function to their clinical intervention. The framework should help the reader organize previously learned information regarding the brain into a more integrated body of knowledge. New information regarding brain functioning will be presented as the framework is outlined, and the reader will be able to conceive of this information within the framework's structure. Finally, the framework will help organize the reader's future acquisition of further information related to brain function in a manner that will optimize the applicability of new information.

Part 1

Basic concepts

Neuropsychological concepts

The application of neuroscience to clinical interventions rests on the premise that different parts of the brain carry out different tasks related to elements of cognition, emotion, and behavior. A client's words and actions during therapy provide information regarding which brain systems are active during therapy and the strengths and weaknesses in these different brain systems. An understanding of underlying brain processes can guide conceptualization of the client's functioning, choices of intervention, and communication with the client during interventions.

Neuropsychology is a field that links observed behaviors to the areas of the brain used in carrying out those behaviors (Lezak, Howieson & Loring, 2004). In its early days, a primary application of neuropsychological assessment involved the use of behavioral observations and tests to help determine the location of damage within the brain. These determinations guided surgical as well as rehabilitation interventions. In recent years, imaging techniques (see Appendix) have been developed that allow non-intrusive examination of brain structure and function, minimizing the need to rely on neuropsychological behavior-based tests for locating brain lesions. However, the idea that specific parts of the brain support specific behaviors remains a powerful guide to understanding the nature of clients' functioning and intervening to help them.

The basic concept underlying neuropsychological assessment is that each behavior relies on activity in a specific set of areas of the brain, and that each area of the brain is involved in only certain types of behavior. If a specific behavior can be carried out successfully, then the areas of the brain needed for the completion of that function can be identified as intact. If a behavior cannot be carried out, then one or more of the areas involved in carrying out that behavior must be impaired. In order to identify brain locations that are the source of specific dysfunction, behavioral tasks can be assigned that use areas of the brain already identified as functioning adequately along with one additional area typically associated with the behavior that can not be completed. Through a process of elimination, the specific area of weakness can be identified.

For example, a particular client's behaviors could be considered with regard to verbal processing, visual–spatial processing, and memory. If a client can easily remember a visual design shown to the client earlier in the day, but has great difficulty remembering a set of words spoken at the same time, it would be suspected that problems with verbal processing are a source of the difficulty. Since the client has shown the ability to remember a visual design, it would be assumed a general memory problem is not the basis of the difficulty remembering the set of words.

The elements of the client's brain being used to produce specific, clinically important behaviors can be considered in light of the stages of processing events and experiences, as well as in light of the contributions of different levels of the brain to understanding and responding to experiences. Stated more succinctly, it is useful to consider the "input–process–output" nature of brain functioning as well as the "top–middle–bottom" influences.

Input–process–output

At the broadest level the brain can be viewed as an information processing system (see Figure 2.1). Data enters the system, the data is processed, and output is generated: input–process–output (Lezak *et al.*, 2004, pp. 18–37). Applying the concepts of neuropsychological assessment,

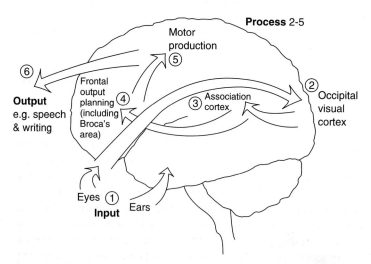

Figure 2.1 Diagram representing input, process, and output of information.

various areas of the brain are used for each stage of information processing, and strengths and weakness in individual areas will shape the manner in which the overall process is carried out.

Input, in this model, includes information gathered through the five senses. It also includes proprioceptive signals initiated by processes active within the body. Sensation is the process whereby stimuli outside the nervous system trigger the firing of receptor neurons in the eyes, ears, nose, skin, or internal tissue that subsequently send neural signals into the brain for processing.

It is useful to imagine a 12-year-old student learning in a classroom. Visual reception systems are activated as he watches what the teacher writes on the chalkboard and observes the pictures and diagrams the teacher displays. Auditory receptors are triggered as he hears his teacher's descriptions of the material. In science class, he may go through the physical steps of carrying out an experiment, thereby activating tactile receptors. As he takes notes, his fingers move and tactile sensory feedback systems associated with writing are stimulated. The olfactory sensory system, evolutionarily the oldest, is less prominent in day-to-day activities such as school, but the student may register the scent of a particular classroom setting, or the pungent smells associated with a science experiment. At the same time that sensory systems deliver information to the brain, neural pathways from internal organs send proprioceptive signals as well, so information regarding the student's physiological state is integrated with other sensory input. In our example of the 12-year-old student, the student's muscles may be tense and his digestive system may be distressed; signals to the brain regarding these states will be encoded along with information from the environment brought in through the various sense organs. At any given moment, reception of current experience consists of an array of stimuli impinging on the student's sensory and proprioceptive systems as information is absorbed.

Processing begins immediately upon reception of input. Multiple areas throughout the brain take part in sorting through incoming information, organizing it, analyzing it, and deciding how to respond (Kandel, Schwartz & Jessell, 2000; Lezak, Howieson & Loring, 2004).

Attention and concentration systems guide other processing systems throughout the brain to become more or less engaged with specific incoming sensory information. Establishing and maintaining attention involves a series of steps including disengaging from the focus of current attention, shifting focus to a new center of attention, amplifying the new focus of attention, and dampening down competing incoming sensory stimuli (Posner & Raichle, 1994). The 12-year-old student in the example will need to attend to the teacher's presentation before he can adequately absorb it and organize it in a way that will be useful in the future. If he is distracted by the girl in the seat next to him he will stop attending to the lesson, and relevant academic material will not be adequately processed.

Perception follows sensation as the brain begins processing incoming information. Signals from individual neurons are combined to yield patterns that are the bases for increasingly complex recognition and understanding. For example, within the visual system the stimulation of individual neurons in the retina of the eye triggers signals that are sent by way of the optic tract to occipital (back of the brain) visual receptive areas (see Figure 2.1). Within the visual cortex the firing of individual neurons progresses from neurons that correspond to specific points on the retina of the eye to neurons in other layers that combine the incoming points of information to yield the perception of specific elements of vision such as points in space, lines, and shapes. These elements are combined to yield a progressively more complete representation of the source of the visual stimulation.

Perception differs from sensation in that the processes occur within the central nervous system rather than at the cells that initially respond to the incoming physical stimulus (Lezak et al., 2004). An implication of the term "perception" is that the integration of information is influenced by the receiver more than is the initial processing at the level of "sensation." This is a difference in relative strength of influence, and it is important to remember that all processing of information by the brain, from sensation to response output, is shaped by characteristics of the brain doing the processing.

Returning to our student trying to pay attention to his teacher rather than to the girl next to him, the words the teacher writes on the board are initially encoded as a series of individual locations on the retina in the back of the eye that fire in response to incoming light. The individual spots associated with the teacher's writing trigger individual neurons in layer IV of the visual cortex in the back of the brain and, in a rapid cascade of firing, are combined from spots to lines to complex shapes as information is passed from layer IV of the visual cortex to layers that combine visual signals in progressively more complex ways. The words put on the chalkboard in front of the student are taking shape in his brain. The visual shapes the student perceives are then sent to cortical association areas at the intersection of the occipital, parietal, and temporal lobes of the brain. In a progressive way, these shapes are recognized as individual symbols (letters), individual symbols are combined into complex symbols (words), complex symbols are combined with meaning, and individual concepts are combined with other concepts in an integration of content, grammar, punctuation, syntax, and context. As part of the process of integration, information travels in from other sensory receptors, such as ears and fingers, in ways similar to the progressive processing of visual information just described. The information from all sensory channels is incorporated into the integration process in the posterior cortical association areas. The student now recognizes what the teacher is saying and writing, and also begins to understand implications and make connections with previous relevant learning.

The output phase follows input and processing. Once recognition and understanding are established, related representations (i.e. neural patterns) in the brain are processed by decision-making centers, many of which are located in the forebrain, and choices are then made regarding actions to be taken in response to the incoming information.

Responses can take a variety of forms, each of which uses a different output system. The student may respond orally by asking a question or making a comment, in which case motor systems related to speech are intentionally activated to express the student's thoughts. The student may write answers to a test, translating his knowledge into highly complex integrated activities associated with handwriting. The student could act out responses in a skit, in which case gross motor processes would be intentionally engaged. The student may respond with facial expressions of interest, boredom, or disgust, whether he is aware of the responses or not. Each of these actions uses parts of the body for expression, and brain signals managing the output rely on different centers and different pathways through the brain. The student may intentionally produce a specific response, for example by writing a thoughtful essay, or may respond without awareness. If the teacher complains he is rolling his eyes in a disgusted way, he may legitimately say to her that he did not know he did it.

During the generation of output, some areas of the brain must be active in order to generate responses in any of several response systems, while other areas of the brain are used only in the production of a response in a particular motor output system. For example, damage to Broca's region in the left frontal quadrant of the cortex interferes with verbal production of both speech and writing (Heilman & Valenstein, 1985), while damage to the area of the motor strip related to speech production would only interfere with the oral production of words (Lezak, Howieson & Loring, 2004 p. 76). Where input can be described as assembling incoming information into progressively more complex organizational units, output can be conceived as moving from a general plan of behavior toward actual behavioral production in progressively more specific units. The final motor pathways our student uses in writing an answer are different from the pathways used to offer an oral response during class discussion.

There are several important characteristics of the brain to consider when analyzing its function during input, process, and output. Breakdown in brain function anywhere along this series of processes will disrupt the input–process–output flow. However, cognitive and behavioral sequelae will vary depending on where the break occurs. A lesion in the visual cortex will interfere with visual perception even though the person's eyes continue to function well. A lesion in regions required for carrying visual representations to the association areas will interfere with integration of visual symbols into verbal functioning. A lesion in the tracts connecting Wernicke's region in posterior integration areas to Broca's region in the frontal lobes on the way to motor production will interfere with the inclusion of meaning in speech even though speech remains possible (Heilman & Valenstein, 1985, p. 30). Furthermore lesions to Broca's region and the motor strip will have effects that have been described in the previous paragraph.

It frequently happens that even though there is a lesion in an area that is involved in a specific aspect of processing, alternative neural pathways may be available that permit some aspect of related processing to continue. Some of these alternate pathways can be intentionally activated. For example, even though areas related to auditory intake may be damaged, processing of verbal meaning through visual perception of words and relationships may permit adequate integration of meaning into both speech and writing. Furthermore, alternate pathways may be used without the awareness of the user. LeDoux demonstrated in rats the presence of direct connections between auditory sensory neurons and central nervous system mechanisms for maintaining a fear response even after connections with the auditory cortex were completely ablated (LeDoux, 1996). Assuming such connections exist in the human brain as well, such connections occur without conscious awareness.

Top–middle–bottom

At the same time that experiences can be considered in terms of the input–process–output flow of information, they can also be considered in terms of various contributions from the "top–middle–bottom" areas of the brain. MacLean (1990) described the levels of the brain from an evolutionary perspective, emphasizing that lower levels of the brain developed earlier in the course of evolution and are relatively simplistic, while higher levels of the brain developed later and are more complex. He also outlined how current experience consists of processing in each of these various levels. Derryberry and Tucker (1992) subsequently described the nature of the contributions of each level of brain functioning to emotional experience, highlighting the reciprocal influence of each level of the brain on other levels.

The brain stem at the "bottom" of the brain regulates the most basic activities, including basic biological processes such as heart rate as well as internal physical states. At the same time, various nuclei, or collections of cells, in the brain stem have direct connections extending throughout the brain. By means of these connections, the brain stem influences responsivity to incoming stimuli of neurons throughout the midbrain and the cortex, where higher levels of cognitive processing occur. There are indications that specific nuclei affect specific areas of the higher levels of the brain, but the specificity of response offered by the brain stem is relatively low (Derryberry & Tucker, 1992). It is useful to think of brain stem influences as turning on and turning off higher level systems in the brain, while activity within the higher levels comprises more finely tuned processing.

There are indications that the ability to successfully manage various specific arousal systems originating in the brain stem develops in conjunction with interactions with caregivers during the early years of life, and that if these early interactions between the infant and the environment are disrupted, management of arousal throughout life will be poor (Schore, 1994). Children suffering early abuse and neglect are likely to have substantial difficulty modulating arousal (De Bellis, 2001; Ford, 2005). As a result, when the surrounding environment is non-stimulating or "boring," the child will tend to shut down. On the other hand, the child will tend to become overly excited or agitated in response to either positive or negative stimulation, with behavioral dyscontrol disrupting interactions with the surrounding environment.

The "middle" area of the brain is focused on the limbic system, including the hippocampus and the amygdala. The level of processing that occurs in the limbic system is more discrete and specific than processing in the brain stem, but not as finely tuned as processing in the cortex (Derryberry & Tucker, 1992). Outputs from the limbic system influence brain stem arousal systems and higher level processing centers in the cortex. "I was so angry I couldn't think straight!" captures the essence of the influence of mid-brain emotional centers on higher order processing. More subtly, these emotion centers in the brain can be viewed as turning on or "priming" areas of the brain supporting complex ideas and memories. In this way, emotion centers influence what thoughts develop in the course of conscious problem-solving.

The cortex at the "top" of the brain provides planning, impulse control, and goal setting necessary for adaptive decision-making and behavior. The cortex is connected to mid-brain and brain stem centers, and by way of these connections, higher-order cognitions can turn on and turn off emotion and arousal centers while also guiding the selection of behaviors to be expressed (Derryberry & Tucker, 1992; Schore, 1994). While an emotion can contribute to the inclination to carry out a specific behavior, for example, punching an adversary, thoughts generated in cortical systems can lead to resisting this impulse after considering potential legal ramifications of such behavior.

As with the "input–process–output" flow of information through the brain, specific "top–middle–bottom" elements of processing depend on functioning of specific centers in the brain and rely on tracts connecting the various parts of the brain (Lezak, Howieson & Loring, 2004). Breakdowns or weak functioning in a specific location will result in specific types of disruption in emotion, cognition, and behavior. Disruption in arousal systems will interfere with thinking and behavior in ways that are different from disruption in cortical systems related to higher order thinking; that is, having a strong impulse uses brain systems that are different from the brain systems used in controlling the impulse. The strength of the impulse and the ability to control expression of the impulse are separate and important elements in generating behavior. Also similar to the "input–process–output" pattern, when there is a breakdown at one level of brain functioning, successful operation at a different level can be activated in order to successfully deal with an experience. For example, if chronic poor control of brain stem arousal systems leads predictably to agitated, impulsive behavior in crowded, poorly structured social settings, a cortex-based decision to avoid the provocative social setting can contribute to maintaining appropriate behavior. Consideration of "top–middle–bottom" elements can thus contribute to both understanding and intervention.

Awareness of the "input–process–output" and "top–middle–bottom" natures of brain functioning can guide psychotherapists to consider a patient's strengths and weaknesses with regard to the type of information being processed, with regard to the various stages in the processing of information, and with regard to the various levels of the brain activated during processing. For example, it may become clear through formal cognitive testing or through informal observation that verbal processing is an area of weakness for a patient while non-verbal processes operate more effectively. In such a case, a patient may respond more effectively through art therapy or psychodrama than through verbal discussion. Similarly, it is possible that social anxiety interferes substantially with oral expression, but private writing remains an available pathway of expression because it eliminates the need to simultaneously integrate awareness of the responses of another person while also developing an appropriate expression of an internal thought or state of emotion. Recognition of the basic steps of processing information in the brain and the levels at which it is processed can organize the psychotherapist's consideration of the patient's strengths and weaknesses.

Five sensory systems plus proprioception contribute to initial perception which leads to higher order processing which is followed by executive decision-making that finally leads to the production of thoughts, emotions, consciously selected behaviors, and behaviors of which the patient remains unaware. Influences at all stages can derive from lower level, generalized brain processes as well as from higher level, fine-tuned analyses. Consideration of the contributions of these steps and levels to the functioning of the patient should help the psychotherapist understand the patient more fully.

3

Neural networks

The previous chapter characterized the brain's processing of experience as a sequential flow of discrete neural events occurring in various locations throughout the brain as information moves from input to output. The description emphasized the "bits and pieces" aspect of brain function. At the same time, the brain's representation of each experience can also be conceived as a single, unique, integrated pattern that includes neurons from widely dispersed areas of the brain (Levine, 2000). Each moment of an experience is a neural network. Each experience is simultaneously bits and pieces of activity and a unified collection of brain processes. The neural network concept provides a framework within which details of various brain processes can be examined. The neural network concept can improve understanding of how individual parts of the brain influence the overall experience of life and how experiences in life are brought to the psychotherapy setting (Vaughan, 1997).

The neural network for any single experience is conceived to be composed of neurons from throughout the brain (see Figure 3.1). Two separate experiences are represented in Figure 3.1, with each experience including neurons from the same areas of the brain, but not sharing individual neurons. The schematic representation includes two sensory areas: an area related to cognitive processing and an area related to processing of emotions. Each individual experience has the potential to include elements from throughout the brain (see to Figure 1.1). Basic arousal systems in the raphe nucleus at the bottom of the brain may be operating in connection with elements of sensory systems in the cortex at the top of the brain, elements of the affect system centered in the amygdala in the mid-section of the brain, frontal decision-making processes, attention focusing systems, motor activation systems in the motor strip, and anxiety modulation areas near the hippocampus. Each experience and each memory are composed of a multitude of neurons firing together at different levels of the brain and in diverse areas. Individual neurons are available to be used in a variety of

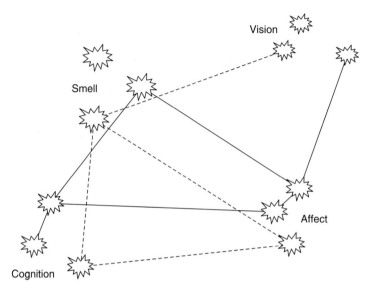

Figure 3.1 Schematic diagram of two neural networks with no shared neurons.

neural networks, with the unique nature of the network being based on the pattern of the neurons involved rather than the fact that a particular neuron is active.

Several aspects of the neural network concept are important to consider. The development of each neural network shapes its subsequent functioning. Once a network is established, activity within a given neural network has basic characteristics that influence how an experience is processed (Table 3.1). Finally, interactions between neural networks influence the processing of new information and the interactions between various memories already stored in the brain (Table 3.1).

Development of neural networks

A specific neural network can be viewed as the culmination of several developments. Genetics guides the construction of basic underlying patterns of connection throughout the brain (Kandel, Schwartz & Jessell, 2000b; Purves & Lichtman, 1985). For example, genetics can lead to one brain emphasizing visual experience while leading another brain to rely more on auditory channels while processing information. Throughout the development of the individual, beginning in utero, interactions with the environment influence the unfolding of genetically guided developmental processes. One brain inclined genetically toward visual processing may,

Table 3.1. Characteristics of neural networks

Characteristics of functioning within networks:
- A memory or experience is based on activity of many individual neurons connected in a network.
- A complete network fires when enough individual neurons in the network fire.
- The neural network is complicated rather than simplistic.
- Connections within networks consist of multiple pathways.
- Multiple brain locations are related to specific functions in a given network.
- Memory uses parts of the brain that were used to encode events.
- Affect is a special and powerful part of neural networks.

Characteristics of functioning between networks:
- Networks share individual neurons.
- Shared neurons lead one network to trigger another.
- Networks compete for level of activity and influence on current brain processing.

through experience, establish multiple neuronal ties between a visual image of mother and a positive feeling of being gratified, while another brain inclined toward visual processing may, through a different set of experiences, connect the visual image of mother with feelings of anguish and lack of gratification. Through repeated experience, synapses that connect various neurons in the network are altered to fire more readily, thereby tying together the pieces of the network. It also appears that connections between neurons of a frequently triggered network are strengthened through the development of an increasing number of synapses connecting each neuron to the others.

Characteristics of individual networks

A network is considered to be activated when a group of neurons associated with a specific experience or memory fires together. A single neuron "fires," that is, sends a signal to another neuron, when it receives enough stimulation from other neurons that its action potential is reached (Kandel, Schwartz & Jessell, 2000b, pp. 19–35). Within the network, the firing of multiple neurons that have experientially been linked in the past will contribute to action potentials being achieved within other neurons in the network; when several neurons in the network fire, they will simultaneously stimulate other neurons in the network, thereby leading those other neurons to fire as well. Eventually, most if not all of the neurons within the network will fire together. For example, input consisting of the smell of autumn leaves combined with the golden glow of the sun at a certain angle can trigger a complete neural network that supports a 30-year-old memory of a college football game shared with a girlfriend wearing a unique brown woven vest.

Experiments related to priming suggest the power of the idea that when enough of the neurons within a network fire, the network will fire more readily. Priming is the process whereby a stimulus is provided that increases the subsequent efficiency or speed with which new information is processed (Posner & Raichle, 1994). A neuron is provided a level of input from other neurons that prepares the neuron to fire, but does not trigger the neuron to fire. In a relevant experiment, if a subject was told to read a list of words and select the ones containing letters written in bold print ("PIANO" versus "PIANO"), parts of the brain related to vision were found to be relatively more active, while if the subject was told to select the words representing manufactured items (PIANO versus APPLE), areas of the brain related to meaning responded more efficiently (Posner & Raichle, 1994, p. 145). Related neurons fire more rapidly when such preparation has been offered. Within the framework of the concept of neural network, a neural network that contains the priming element has been stimulated ahead of time and, when other elements of the network are presented later, it reaches threshold for firing more rapidly than if priming had not occurred. Priming may be done by offering a concept to guide processing (Posner & Raichle, 1994), by providing a list of words that are part of the network of interest (Graf *et al.*, 1984), or by evoking mood or emotion that is part of the network (LeDoux, 1996; Zajonc, 1980). Each of these manners of priming the network makes it more likely that activities related to the priming stimulus will occur more rapidly.

Variations in therapy intervention can be conceived as variations in the manner in which relevant neural networks exist and are activated. Psychodynamic transference can be conceived as a way in which previously developed neural networks characterizing a person's relationships are used in a current relationship. Experiences during the therapy relationship have elements that are also part of neural networks created during previous relationship experiences, and old neural networks are triggered by current experiences and become available for conscious consideration. Gestalt interventions focus on using multisensory experiences that are assumed to access important neuronal networks and then lead to new experiences that can add to or shift the old network. Functional exposure in behavior therapy habituation interventions can be considered to activate maladaptive networks and then maintain connection with these networks while the affective elements of the network stop firing. At the end of the exposure time this yields a connection with an inactive affect system that will be recalled outside the therapy setting because connections within the neural network have been shifted.

Connections within a network vary in ways that add complexity to the system. Connections between some neurons build through a basic pairing process whereby repeated, simultaneous, joint firing of two neurons strengthens the synapses joining them (Kandel, Schwartz & Jessell, 2000b, pp. 1247–79). Connections between other neurons are built on complex integration that occurs in association areas that bring together and combine many types of information from many areas of the brain (Vaughan, 1997). Many of the interconnecting systems in the brain are founded on inhibitory processes whereby firing of one neuron inhibits the firing of another neuron while facilitating the firing of yet another (Kandel, Schwartz & Jessell, 2000b, pp. 26–7 & 205–28; Posner & Raichle, 1994, p. 149). Thus, the experience of a specific memory may be based on the inhibition of neurons as well as on the activation of other neurons. For example, the similarities between the loss of a current lover and the previous loss of a mothering figure may lead to sudden and complete connections between the two experiences. As a consequence, the loss of the lover begins to evoke much greater feelings of loss than the particular parting warrants. Alternately, the similarity between the current break up and a previous loss may generate such strong and inhibiting anxiety that the memory of the new separation is severely disrupted to the point that subsequent recall of the recent event is severely impaired.

Neural networks are likely to be connected by way of multiple pathways. Some pathways are likely to include areas of the cortex that are available to conscious processes, while other pathways are likely to be through subcortical tracts that offer little likelihood of being consciously identified. LeDoux (1996) conducted research with rats that helped identify a sub-cortical neural pathway between auditory receptor cells and the amygdala, which houses a primary center in the brain for processing fear. It was originally believed that auditory input must pass from auditory receptors through the auditory processing center in the cortex and then to the amygdala in order for fear learning to be established. LeDoux first trained rats to expect electrical shock whenever a bell sounded. Later, all connections between auditory receptor neurons and the cortex were cut. Experimental rats continued to respond to a bell with signs of fear after the connections were cut. It was discovered that this response remained due to the activity of a previously unidentified subcortical pathway. If a human subject experienced the same removal of cortical connections after developing a classically conditioned association between sound and shock, the subject would continue to demonstrate fear when the bell sounded; however, the human subject would report being baffled regarding why the fear was occurring. Such a fear response to sound might then remain unexplained no matter how many years of psychoanalysis the subject subsequently obtained.

Considered in this light, asking the question "Why did you do it?" becomes suspect since inputs to the motor system carrying out a behavior likely include a greater or lesser number of inputs to which the individual can never obtain conscious access. Each network activated likely includes elements accessible to conscious thought as well as elements beyond the reach of direct, conscious reflection. A client's verbal explanation of "why" the client takes specific actions will only account for a portion of the neural inputs to the motor system that produced the observed behavior.

Each neural network consists of elements scattered throughout the brain. Referring to Figure 1.1, a network may include frontal lobe decision making processes, attention focusing, visual and auditory sensory systems, associated emotions and levels of arousal, and motor responses. Various activities have been found to be associated with activity in different areas of the brain, and a network related to a specific type of activity will not activate all areas of the brain equally.

Specific locations in the brain are dedicated to carrying out specific tasks. This does not mean that a specific place in the brain independently functions to support a single phenomenologically individual experience. Rather, specific locations carry out tasks in conjunction with myriad other areas carrying out their tasks in a coordinated manner. Loss of one center in the brain may lead to the whole pattern breaking down, or to the pattern shifting somewhat in nature. As an example, centers have been identified that are necessary for the identification of emotion in facial expression (Bowers et al., 1993). The absence of functioning in this area can lead to a person having understanding of emotions without the ability to identify emotions when they are expressed on the faces of others. In another example, if Broca's area (a frontal lobe center for guiding the initiation of speech) is damaged, a person may have capacities to assemble words yet be unable to form those words into spoken speech. The use of multiple individual areas to produce a single response has two primary implications. First, an individual neural network pattern will be affected by what brain systems are structurally available. Second, it will be affected by what systems are functionally active or shut down due to patterns of stimulation or inhibition within the network. Anxiety associated with fear of rejection may lead to functional impairment of the facial recognition system even though the necessary physical structure within the individual is intact. However, the facial recognition system may, through the interaction of genetics and experience, be so poorly developed physically that the person cannot include it in the neural networks that develop in the course of processing information.

Memory has been found to use the primary cortical sensory areas to store elements of a memory related to that sensory system (Kandel, Kupferman & Iverson, 2000a; Zubicaray et al., 2001). When a neural network yields a visual memory, the visual sensory cortex is being activated in conjunction with other areas of the brain more commonly considered to be centers of memory. Such a model offers understanding of the nature of flashbacks experienced by victims of traumatic events. During a flashback the visual system is activated as part of the traumatic memory and, as a result, the visual system is not available for use in reception of new visual input. Neural networks associated with the memory of a traumatic event include a high level of emotional intensity derived from emotion centers in the amygdala (LeDoux, 1996; McGaugh, 2004). This intensity gives "power" to the flashback, and this power effectively prevents frontal lobe executive centers from intentionally using the visual system to process current input. As a result, a client may experience a temporary inability to see the external environment even though frontal, decision-making areas of the brain are attempting to override the control over visual processing exerted by the powerful flashback. If a client understands the reason he cannot see the therapist while experiencing the flashback, the likelihood that the client will view himself as "crazy" will be lower.

Recognition that sensory input systems are used during re-creation of sensations in a memory implies, within the construct of the neural network, how external sensory input can trigger a particular memory. When enough sensory neurons involved in current visual perception are also part of a previously stored memory, the neural network associated with the memory reaches the point that the whole network fires and the memory is recalled. This is true for flashbacks as well as for day-to-day memories.

Affect appears to be a special and powerful element within a neural network. Emotion has been shown to be closely intertwined with memory (McGaugh, 2004), and may actually be considered to be a poorly refined but important and powerful element of memory that can stimulate action without the individual taking time to consciously assess the stimulus in a more conscious and systematic manner (LeDoux, 1996). Affect has been described as changing higher order processing through a bottom-to-top influencing mechanism (Derryberry & Tucker, 1992). There are indications that connections between affect and sensory experience continue to be established even when higher order integration systems shut down due to the influences of stress and trauma (LeDoux, 1996). Affect within a neural network is therefore likely to be resistant to influence by higher order thought processes at times because neural pathways connecting higher order thought to emotion are likely to be limited.

In the present model, affect is conceived to strongly influence the activation of the neural network. A specific emotion is likely to be connected to a variety of experiences, and the emotion likely triggers occurrence of related neural networks even when numbers of shared sensory neurons is low. It seems likely that metaphor, within and outside therapy, works by activating neural networks even though literal connections (Coulson & Van Petten, 2002) or sensory similarities are minimal. Affect seems likely to be a primary connector supporting the influence of disparate metaphors on thematically similar material. Asking clients to experience an emotion and then notice what thoughts pop into their heads is a strategy that can lead to identification of connections between apparently unrelated experiences. Activating affect may also be critical in order to carry out a variety of therapeutic change interventions. If a client can be helped to observe the experience of affect within a setting in which the affect is incongruent, the incongruence of the affect can be more readily influenced by higher order decision-making mechanisms. Basic processes of habituation and sensitization in individual neurons have been described by Kandel (2000) and seem likely to be active in the development and change of affective contributions to the neural network. Recognizing and understanding these processes can guide development of appropriate interventions.

Network interactions

Several characteristics of connections between networks are important to consider along with characteristics of within-network activity. Characteristics of interconnection have been implied in the previous discussion of characteristics of neurons firing within networks, but they should be directly considered in order to fully understand the effects of neural networks on personal experience and processes that occur in therapy. Networks share individual neurons. The more similar one network is to another network, the more likely it is that activation of one network will activate another network. Finally, networks "compete"; that is, if one network is active, other networks are less likely to be active.

It was previously pointed out that each experience is based on activity in a network composed of multiple individual neurons; an individual experience is not based on the activity of a single neuron. The essence of the network concept is not that each neuron or each part of the brain has a specific memory, but that each memory is the experience of a unique combination of scattered individual neurons that also participate in many other networks (see Figure 3.2). The two experiences schematically represented in Figure 4.1 share neurons in each of the four activity areas depicted. It may be that two networks are extremely similar and share neurons in similar if not identical areas of the brain. For example, hearing two different lectures by different teachers about the same topic may activate neurons in the same areas of the brain. It is also frequently the case that one network that shares neurons with another network contains neurons in areas that are not activated by the second network. For example,

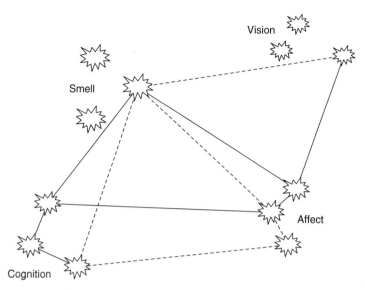

Figure 3.2 Schematic diagram of two neural networks sharing neurons.

a student may hear information about the battle of the Alamo from his teacher and he may read information about the Alamo in a book. Networks related to these two means of gathering information about the Alamo will share many neurons, but one network will include neurons in visual cortex related to reading while the other will include neurons in auditory cortex related to hearing the teacher.

Characteristics of within-network activity previously described help explain the effects one network is likely to have on another. The more similar one network is to another, the more neurons there are in the second network that fire when the first network fires, and the more likely it is that the second network will reach the threshold at which the complete second network fires. One experience or memory thus triggers another. The stronger the connections are that exist between neurons shared by the two networks and non-shared neurons in the second network, the more likely the first network is to trigger the second network. Strength of connection may be related to the number of neurons connected or to a history of frequent mutual firing that has resulted in the establishment of very strong connections between just a few neurons. Shared emotions are considered to be especially likely to trigger other networks because they are a central part of memory and because they have the potential to form strong connections with neurons in other areas of the brain during meaningful life experiences.

In a previous example, autumn scents and hues of sunlight were described as triggering memories of a college girlfriend. Remembered images of the girlfriend may then trigger other memories of the same girlfriend in settings having no connection to autumn smells or golden sun. These subsequent memories may elicit recollections of heartache and loss in a totally different physical setting in one's past. In this example, an initial triggering stimulus activated a specific neural network that then activated a cascade of networks as one network triggered another through shared neurons related to non-visual sensations, visual images, and emotion.

Current experiences that are similar to old experiences will trigger the old patterns to fire, and these old patterns are likely to influence the brain's processing of the new situation. Neurons firing at the top, middle, and bottom areas of the brain all influence each other (Derryberry & Tucker, 1992). Emotions that are part of the old experience may be powerful enough to strongly influence the processing of the new experience. If a person has experienced repeated painful interpersonal betrayals throughout childhood, then the slightest hint of disregard displayed by the current spouse will trigger strong emotions related to fear of betrayal that lead to the person misinterpreting the current spouse as being ready to leave – even though the reality is that the current spouse is simply being somewhat self-preoccupied.

Furthermore, the conscious experience associated with the firing of a given neural network is likely only a small aspect of the network. Many processes within a specific network occur subcortically (LeDoux, 1996) and therefore without conscious awareness. It may therefore be that connections within and between networks can be better intuited through understanding the various brain processes involved than through noticing the conscious, face-valid elements of the experience.

There is evidence to suggest that in addition to triggering similar neural networks, neural networks compete with other networks for activation. Posner and Raichle (1994, p. 149) pointed out that when a person is prompted to attend to a prime, that is, to a particular type of target stimulus, then responses in the brain to unrelated targets are slowed. This suggests that an active network operating more effectively than one that is less active is more likely to engage areas of the brain related to conscious awareness. It seems likely that whether attention to a target is triggered by instructions provided by an experimenter or by a high level of similarity between current and past experiences, once attention is drawn to a network, the network becomes increasingly likely to be the network of which a person is aware. For example, if a person is driving down the road talking on a cellular telephone, the person is likely to have the experience of not being conscious of passing a particular landmark even though the person drove the car past the location. Networks consciously attended to during the conversation precluded awareness of networks related to visually processing the landmark. This example also highlights the fact that neural networks outside the realm of conscious awareness remain active, since networks related to driving the car must have been active even though the driver was not attending to those networks and related external experiences. Another example of one network taking over a person's experience and blocking out a competing network would be the previously offered description of an abuse victim's flashback in the therapist's office preventing the patient from being able to see the therapist.

Consideration of neural networks as patterns of neurons throughout the brain connected in various ways begins to shift the understanding of the relationship between a person's phenomenological experience and the underlying brain processes that support that phenomenology. Some of the connections between neurons are very simple. Associationistic connections between pairs of neurons at different levels of the brain demonstrate the power of repetition to shift what a person is likely to think, whether the person is aware of the associations being made or not. Other connections between neurons are very complicated. The hippocampus receives stimulation from multiple areas of the brain, interconnections between pyramidal cells within the hippocampus are extremely complex, and the process of long-term potentiation (see Chapter 4) contributes to the rapid development of new connections that support complex reasoning and new insights. Whether simple or complex, the ways these connections operate are far removed from the logic we use during conscious analysis of problems. The powerful impact of subcortical neurons on the activity of higher level neurons implies the presence of influences on thinking occurring far below conscious awareness, and brings into focus the difference between dynamic conceptualizations of the unconscious and the unconscious processes operating in our brains independent of processes of repression or other psychological defenses.

The combined concepts of stepwise processing of information and the presence of neural networks that include neurons throughout the brain provide a context within which several important brain systems and processes can be considered. Variations in types of learning and memory appear to rely on different areas and activities in the brain identified in Figure 1.1. Figure 1.1 also identifies areas of the brain related to affect (emotion) and anxiety. Not represented in the figure is the powerful influence of brain development on what brain systems are available to process information at specific stages of development, and how developmental level affects the nature of neural networks that are established at various stages of development. Each of these will be considered in subsequent chapters.

4

Memory and learning

Memory can be defined as the process whereby "knowledge is encoded, stored, and later retrieved" (Kandel *et al.*, 2000a, p. 1245). On its surface, such a definition hints the brain is a static recording device waiting to take in and store the input offered to it. This is not the case. Instead, the brain interacts with the environment, including the external world and the person's own body, in multiple dynamic ways and changes form in response to these interactions. The form the brain takes subsequently influences its interactions with the environment in the future. Stated another way, "Memory is thus the way the brain is affected by experience and then subsequently alters its future responses" (Siegel, 1999, p. 24). Psychotherapy can be viewed as a process of recognizing how the brain has been shaped by its past and then applying this recognition to develop better ways to use the brain in future interactions with the world.

Memory can be viewed at various levels, each of which can offer different insights into human function. Global effects of experience on brain development can be viewed as one aspect of memory. Intracellular processes have been identified that support various memory processes. Connections between cells support memory in several ways, each of which offers its own implications for the development and maintenance of memories. Important processes related to intercellular connection include the strengthening of individual connections, long-term potentiation, habituation, and sensitization. Different types of memory systems appear to be at work throughout the brain, supporting significantly different types of memory and learning. For the purposes of the present conceptualization, biochemical processes within cells will not be addressed (see Kandel *et al.*, 2000b, pp. 1247–79). The other aspects of memory mentioned will each be described.

Brain development itself can be considered a form of memory to the extent that experience alters the shape of the brain and therefore the way it perceives and reacts to incoming stimulation. Experiments with rats (Bennett *et al.*, 1964) and cats (Hubel & Wiesel, 1970) have revealed changes in cortical weight and structure based on early experience. Children who have not been exposed to language before adolescence have been found to have permanent deficits in their ability to develop language (Newport, 1990). The areas of the brain needed for processing language have not developed in the absence of appropriate experiences, and the difficulty learning language can be considered to be an expression of the brain's memory of the early deprivation. This is not a traditional way of conceptualizing memory, but it highlights the profound influence of experience on the brain and thereby on human behavior even when the early experience itself is not in conscious awareness. A client enters psychotherapy with a brain and related capacities and deficits molded by previous experiences.

Intercellular processes

The basic feature of intercellular memory processes is that neurons become paired with each other (Kandel *et al.*, 2000b, pp. 1254–7). When two connecting neurons fire at the same time, they are more likely to fire again in the future because the strength of the connections between them will be stronger. The strength of the signal sent through an individual synapse connecting the two neurons will become stronger over the course of repeated experience. In addition, it appears that when two connected neurons fire frequently together, they may develop new synaptic boutons, which are points of connection, and thereby increase even more the likelihood that when the sending neuron fires, the receiving neuron will also reach its action potential and fire as well. These memory processes seem likely to be the basis for implicit, procedural, or non-hippocampal learning that will be discussed in the 'Memory Systems' section of this chapter. A prominent implication of such learning is that simple repetition can effect change, even in the absence of reasoning or logic to support the change. One way that change occurs in therapy is that previous fear, hurt, or loneliness is experienced in the presence of an emotionally supportive relationship rather than in the presence of abandonment. After multiple repetitions, vulnerability becomes associated with the experience of emotional support, and then both experiences occur where before only the fear and abandonment occurred. The person is then less overwhelmed by triggers that once left them powerless.

A more complicated intercellular pattern of connection appears to support memory identified as explicit memory, which is based in the hippocampus and affiliated brain structures. Long term potentiation (Kandel *et al.*, 2000b, pp. 1259–64) is a process in which two previously unrelated neurons can be associated in a way that supports new ways of integrating information (see Figure 4.1). When two neurons (A and B) both enervate a third neuron (C), the process of long term potentiation can in effect form a bond between them even though they are not directly connected. If neurons A and B fire at the same time, leading to neuron C firing, the bonds between C and each of the other neurons is strengthened. In the future, either one of the neurons A or B is more likely to be able to cause C to fire independently. Whereas previously only one neuron (A) could cause C to fire, now either A or B can cause C to fire, so a new memory is supported.

Pyramidal cells (neurons that receive input from extremely high numbers of other neurons) are structured in a way that facilitates development of such new connections. These cells occur in high numbers in the hippocampus. They have multiple incoming receptors and are therefore particularly amenable to such learning. Connections between the hippocampus and frontal cortical areas appear to support conscious processing and decision making, and the area as a whole is particularly well designed to establish novel connections supporting new learning. Such a set of connections may support change in the therapy setting. If a person experienced abuse by males in early life, then working with a male therapist offers a new connection. Interaction with the therapist triggers trust, and the concept of male, which previously did not trigger trust, comes to do so because it occurs at the same time that therapy with a male occurs. Whereas the associative processes outlined earlier support the process of strengthening

Action potential

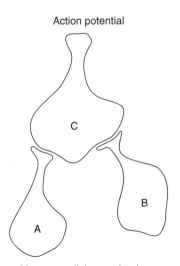

Memory: cellular mechanisms

Figure 4.1 Three cells arranged to support long term potentiation.

previous connections, the three cell long term potentiation model supports the development of new connections – implying new ways of experiencing life.

Kandel has offered models of intercellular connection that can support the development of habituation and sensitization to stimuli from the external world (Kandel *et al.*, 2000b, pp. 1248–52). These models have the potential to guide conceptualization of the processing of emotional material. Repeated stimulation of sensory cells in the absence of other arousal or provocation has been observed to lead to habituation, that is, to reduced likelihood that the sensory stimulation will lead to the previously automatic behavioral response. This offers a model at the level of intercellular activity of how habituation to fear might occur, and it supports repeated continuous exposure to a negative stimulus in order to help a client become less reactive to previously painful experiences. Such a model is clearly applicable to exposure treatments for phobia, but may also apply to more complex painful emotional experiences confronted in more complicated psychotherapy situations.

Kandel and his associates have also demonstrated an intercellular model whereby an organism can be sensitized to experiences with the environment. A noxious stimulus presented to one sensory neuron of the organism heightens the responsiveness of other sensory neurons as well as the motor neurons they activate. In this way, the connection between the sensory neuron and the motor neuron can be substantially strengthened so that the reaction is stronger and more resistant to habituation. This model suggests a basis for the resistance to improvement observed in cases of Post Traumatic Stress Disorder. If the face of a bearded man has been paired with the extreme emotional and physical pain of a rape, it may be very difficult for the victim to stop reacting strongly and negatively to any person with a beard.

Consideration of the models of habituation and sensitization seems likely to offer eventual insight into the processes involved in recovering from traumatic experiences. However, it is unclear now whether abreactive or exposure therapies are likely to sensitize the person to the negative experience, thereby prolonging and intensifying the debilitating negative reactions involved, or are likely to lead to habituation if exposure is maintained for an extended period of time.

Memory systems

Current conceptualizations of memory systems have divided memory into at least two general types of processes, and these processes appear to rely on different parts of the brain for their implementation. One conceptualization divides memory processes into explicit and implicit memory, while another divides memory into declarative and non-declarative memory. While not identical in their differentiations, declarative and explicit memories are similarly conceptualized as learning that includes or is available to conscious awareness and narrative explanation, while implicit and non-declarative memories are viewed as occurring outside of awareness and being much less available to conscious, narrative influence (Schacter & Tulving, 1994, p. 25).

O'Keefe and Nadel (1978) focused on the differences between learning that involved the hippocampal system and learning that did not. Hippocampal learning appears to coincide with declarative and explicit conceptualizations of learning, while non-hippocampal learning appears to coincide with implicit memory formation.

Damage to the hippocampus impairs or eliminates the ability to learn new information in a conscious way. In one example of the effects of damage to explicit memory systems, a female client met with a specific doctor each day over an extended period of time. Each time she met with the doctor she had to be reintroduced to him since she had no conscious memory of the previous meetings. However, the doctor began holding a sharp pin in his hand each day as he shook hands upon meeting the client. After several visits, the client would refuse to shake the doctor's hand even though she professed no memory of previously meeting the doctor, and could not offer a reason for her reluctance to shake the doctor's hand (LeDoux, 1996, pp. 180–2). It seems likely the loss of hippocampal functioning resulted in the client losing the capacity for formation of conscious, narrative memories. However, she maintained the ability to learn to associate fear with a repeated painful event, as well as the ability to alter her behavior when confronted with the same event later. The implication of this example is that clients learn many things of which they are unaware even though the things learned shape their behavior significantly. Emotional learning, which is particularly relevant to the process of psychotherapy, is characterized by such learning.

The hippocampus and associated brain structures appear to support the development of relational or spatial maps within which incoming information can be understood. Research with rats running mazes has found that once a normal rat has become familiar with a maze and has developed a route by which it can reach a reward, if the route is altered, the rat can relatively quickly develop an alternative pathway for reaching the goal. If the rat has had the hippocampus rendered non-functional, it can learn to follow a pathway to the reward but, if the pathway is altered, the animal has a very difficult time finding a successful alternative pathway to the reward (O'Keefe & Nadel, 1979; Tsien et al., 1996). There are indications that similar problems exist with regard to developing new strategies for reaching goals in situations that are not based on visual spatial relationships (Squire *et al.*, 1993). It thus appears that the hippocampus is an important piece in the development of concepts that guide our problem-solving, while it remains possible to learn through rote rehearsal even in the absence of involvement of the hippocampus.

The hippocampus and nearby cortical regions receive input from throughout the brain (Squire, 1992) (see Figure 4.2). Specific sources of input include sensory systems, perceptual systems, association areas within sensory areas of the cortex, areas of association between various sensory areas of the brain, and areas of the cortex physically adjacent to the hippocampus, including the cingulate and the frontal lobes. The hippo-campus is therefore well-suited to serve as an integration area that supports novel conceptualizations and the memory of such insights.

O'Keefe and Nadel (1978) identified the following characteristics of hippocampal learning:
- All or none
- Rapid acquisition and extinction
- Motivated by exploration and novelty
- Less prone to interference
- Focuses on unique elements

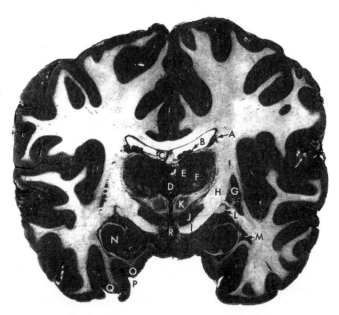

Figure 4.2 Coronal view of the brain with the hippocampus located at N. (with permission, from Watson, 1995.)

- Flexible
- Gives context

These characteristics support efficient processing of incoming information and integration of new information with information previously stored in the brain. They also support flexible retrieval of stored information. However, these characteristics do not support the establishment of a rigid, permanent record of events experienced.

It is conceived that within the explicit memory system the hippocampus and other closely associated brain structures support the formation and storage of memories within a context (Jacobs & Nadel, 1998). The hippocampus and associated structures provide the context, but specific elements are stored throughout the brain. Retrieval of explicit memories involves the "re-aggregation" of the various individual elements within a contextual structure, and this re-aggregation is experienced as an episodic memory that is often available to the individual for conscious consideration. This re-aggregation is very different from pushing a button and watching the replay of an event recorded earlier. Rather, the re-aggregation is a constructive event, and as such is influenced by the state of the brain at the time the memory is recalled. The memory process is therefore vulnerable to disruption.

Explicit memories can be influenced at the point of encoding as well as during recall (Okado & Stark, 2005). Research into false memories has demonstrated that explicit memories may shift due to disrupted encoding of information related to specific facts or related to the context within which the fact is received. Level and type of emotion a person experiences can influence both encoding and recall (McGaugh, 2004). False memory research has provided evidence that characteristics of encoding such as length of exposure to original input can influence the stability of memories (Loftus, 2005) and that as time passes from the initial encoding of information, the information becomes more vulnerable to being changed based on external influences (Loftus & Hoffman, 1989). Jacobs and Nadel (1998) suggested that autobiographical memory, that is, our conscious memory of an event, "is produced through the re-aggregation of dispersed information and a 'filling in' or 'smoothing out' accomplished through inferential processes." It is therefore important to remember that even though explicit memories may seem solid, they are creations rather than recordings.

While the hippocampus, in concert with nearby cortical areas and frontal lobe centers, plays a central role in initially organizing and subsequently retrieving explicit memories, it is not the location in the brain in which long-term memories are stored (Wiltgen et al., 2004). Rather, it appears that for an extended period of time the hippocampus supports the maintenance of memory traces that include information stored in the frontal lobes (prefrontal cortex), associative cortical areas, and primary sensory cortical areas such as visual cortex. Over time the location of coordination of memory maintenance shifts from the hippocampus to a collection of centers including areas of the prefrontal cortex, the temporal cortices on either side of the brain, and cortical association centers in the parietal area identified in the upper, back portions of the brain (see Figure 1.1). This shift in location of mechanisms of memory maintenance and coordination accounts for the fact that when the hippocampus and closely related areas are damaged, recent memories are lost but memories of the distant past are maintained (Squire, 1992).

Another characteristic of explicit memory systems is that primary sensory cortical areas are used in memory as well as during initial perception of information (Farah, 1989; Weinberger, 2004). The center of coordination of a given memory may shift from the hippocampus to other brain sites over time as the memory is established in long term memory, but it appears that the primary sensory cortices remain active participants in initial and long term memory processes. Furthermore, the primary sensory cortices that are highly involved in hippocampal, explicit memory (Wiltgen et al., 2004) also play a central role in implicit memory (Squire, 1992).

While explicit, declarative memory appears to consist of a relatively well-organized set of processes, the concept of implicit memory includes a variety of types of learning that appear to rely on direct pairing of simultaneously active, connected neurons (Kandel et al., 2000b, pp. 1247–59). If one neuron reaches an action potential, and then a neuron to which it sends a signal also reaches an action potential, the connection between those two neurons becomes stronger, and the likelihood that the second neuron will fire when the first one does is increased. The increased likelihood of firing is learning. Procedural memory, defined as the memory of steps of a task, works through repeated rehearsal whereby a first step is followed repeatedly by a second step which is followed by a third step, and so forth, to the point that the steps begin to follow one after the other in a much more rapid sequence.

Other implicit memories may include associating two independent stimuli that occur simultaneously. The learning in this case may not involve a task to be completed; rather, it may involve learning of the connection between words and parts of words (Graf et al., 1984; Squire, 1992). Studies conducted by Squire and his associates have demonstrated the presence of such learning even when hippocampal systems have been severely damaged through stroke or cerebral event. In these studies subjects were shown a list of words and were later asked to recall the words in the list. When the subjects were prompted to recall the words from the previously learned list, those with hippocampal damage performed much more poorly than normal subjects. When the subjects were given word stems and asked to use the word stems to help remember words from the previous list, the brain damaged subjects again did much worse than the normal subjects. However, when subjects were instructed to say the first word that came to mind after being exposed to a word stem, brain injured and normal subjects performed equally well. This finding was interpreted to reflect the presence of priming, which is considered to be implicit, associative learning that occurred even though the person could not intentionally remember the word list effectively. It is suggestive of unconscious processes that support the activation of neural networks underlying the emergence of new material during the psychotherapy process.

Research indicates that development of associations between events and emotions is an example of non-hippocampal learning based on simple pairing, even in the absence of awareness and insight. LeDoux (1996) described the process whereby in the presence of severe trauma, the hippocampal system ceases to function effectively. That is, aware learning and memory is disrupted. However, he indicated that memories associating fear with incoming sensory information are made even stronger by the same neuro-chemical events that disrupt hippocampal functioning. The result is that a subject can learn to be afraid of something without being consciously aware of the experience that is being learned. His research with rats revealed that a learned fear reaction to a sound will be maintained by an animal even after all connections between the ear and the cortex are destroyed. He and his colleagues discovered that subcortical neural connections exist leading from auditory sensory cells to the amygdala. This suggests that people can learn to associate a stimulus with negative affect even if they are unaware of the event occurring.

O'Keefe and Nadel (1978) described non-hippocampal learning as having the following characteristics:
- Incremental
- Slow acquisition and extinction
- Focus on categories not concepts
- More prone to interference
- Focus on similarities
- Rigid, non-flexible
- Category, not context

The differences between hippocampal and non-hippocampal learning suggest that insight has separate and very different effects than repeated experience has on changing what has been learned in the past. It seems likely that insight based on hippocampal learning processes offers the chance to quickly develop new ways of looking at information, and thereby offers a good means of adapting to new situations (Wiltgen et al., 2004). However, it also seems likely that neuronal connections based on implicit, non-hippocampal learning will not readily change despite the presence of new insight. Expressed neuronally, a particular pattern of input or past experience may become paired with new ideas and concepts through hippocampal learning and long-term potentiation. However, past neuronal associations developed through intense experience or repeated rehearsal are likely to remain strong despite the presence of insight that would argue to the contrary.

The lack of synchrony between these two forms of learning can be very distressing for clients who believe that continuing to have maladaptive emotional reactions despite the presence of insight to the contrary is evidence of the severity and permanence of their pathology. The lack of synchrony leaves clients feeling very out of control of themselves in a basic way that threatens self-esteem and positive identity. When implicit memory associations weaken, they are likely to do so slowly and incrementally over time. This appears to be particularly likely to be the case in situations involving strong emotional reactions. LeDoux (1996) has proposed that hippocampal memory processes may develop insightful memory of previous emotional trauma by adding affect to conscious memory through "developing a memory of the memory." Conceived in this way, hippocampal memory begins to include non-hippocampal memory in a fuller integration that adds emotion to conscious conceptualization, thereby combining new frontal lobe analysis with basic sensory and affective schema from the past.

The concept of "infantile amnesia" is illuminated when considering the differences between hippocampal and non-hippocampal memory systems. Long-term memory storage that includes hippocampal memory systems does not come "on line" until around the age of 3 or 4 years old. It appears that even after the hippocampus begins to develop and becomes available for integration of incoming information, cortical areas influenced by the hippocampus and apparently required for long-term memory storage remain undeveloped for a period of time (Squire *et al.*, 1993). Hence, learning that occurs prior to that time will not typically be available to explicit, narrative memory. Instead, the child has stored early experiences in implicit memory systems which are operating during the earliest months of life. Following the reasoning offered by LeDoux (1996), it seems likely that sometimes a person can become aware of sensory memories and connected affect stored during these early years; conscious "memory of the memory" may then mediate awareness of such early experiences. However, it also seems likely that such memories will not be the same as memories stored using hippocampal systems later in life.

Considering memory from the cellular level to the level of memory systems provides an integrated appreciation for the processes that formed the client prior to entering therapy as well as the processes whereby the client changes. Simple repeated pairing of neurons throughout the brain has contributed to the development of stronger synapses and greater numbers of synapses supporting the particular neural networks the client brings to therapy. Simple neuronal synaptic pairings help explain the patterns of strength and weakness in the client's ability to interact with the environment.

During therapy, new and hopefully more adaptive experiences slowly build new patterns of strength and weakness in synaptic function whereby new patterns of adaptive coping can be established. At the level of the single cell, repeated sensory firing in the presence of intense arousal has likely resulted in increased rate of firing in response to relatively low levels of arousal; the client has likely become sensitized to specific experiences in ways that are unique to that client. However, if the client has had repeated experiences in the absence of significant arousal, habituation has likely occurred whereby there is little likelihood of response to a specific stimulus, so some stimuli or situations are likely to seem irrelevant to the particular client. Upon entering therapy, the occurrence of previously arousing events in a setting that reduces the intense arousal can lead to reduced likelihood the neuron will fire in the future; clients can habituate to historically negative experiences if sensory stimuli occur without the negative consequences.

All of these processes support learning and memory in implicit memory systems as well as in explicit memory systems. Long-term potentiation occurring primarily in the hippocampus supports the rapid establishment of new neural connections in explicit memory, and these explicit connections support awareness, insight, and opportunities for change in the context of psychotherapy. Finally, recognizing the disparate natures of implicit versus explicit processing of information allows appreciation of the nature of the inconsistencies that regularly occur in the ways clients experience themselves and in the ways they behave.

The broad conceptualizations of input–process–output and neural networks rest on the basic processes of memory. Incoming information can be incorporated through the strengthening of individual synapses connecting two neurons in implicit memory as well as through complex integration processing in the hippocampus using long-term potentiation in the establishment of explicit memory. Neural networks include complex conscious insights founded on the integration within the hippocampus of information from throughout the brain. Neural networks also include the implicit connecting of pairs of cells far below the level of conscious processing. Recognition of these various ways in which the brain manages the experiences of life can shift the views of therapists as well as clients during the course of psychotherapy.

The particularly important role of affect was highlighted in the chapter on neural networks. It was also noted that memory is highly influenced by affect (McGaugh, 2004). Having delineated in a basic way the brain processes underlying memory, it is then useful to consider the influence of emotion on how the memory systems and the brain as a whole work.

5

Affect

The previously presented description of the neural network concept briefly identified the special contributions of affect to neural network patterns and to memory processes. The connections between affect and memory should be clearly delineated.

The amygdala (see Figure 1.1) is a primary center for the processing of emotions (LeDoux, 2002; McGaugh, 2004). Multiple connections exist between the amygdala and the hippocampus, and there is strong evidence that the two areas of the brain work in tandem. LeDoux (1996) has suggested that hippocampal integrations would be affect-free without the connections between the amygdala and the hippocampus. However, the amygdala also has direct and indirect interconnections with sensory cortex and sensory receptor neurons, so ties between sensory information and emotion can be established both with and without conscious awareness and explicit memory systems (LeDoux, 1996).

It appears that the amygdala contributes to memory storage by activating memory consolidation processes in other parts of the brain when positive or negative emotion is present (McGaugh, 2004). Stimuli with positive or negative emotional valence are remembered more clearly than are neutral stimuli. For example, faces with either positive or negative expressions are remembered better than are faces with neutral expressions, and neural imaging of the brain indicates that increased amygdala activity accompanied by commensurate hippocampal activity parallels the differences in learning (Dolcos *et al.*, 2003). Neutral stimuli are learned more effectively, as well, when followed by administration or stimulation of hormones or neurotransmitters associated with emotion and activation of the amygdala. Multiple studies of the effects of various patterns of activation and deactivation of areas of the brain have demonstrated that specific subsections of the amygdala uniquely facilitate the observed modulation of memory for emotional information in the hippocampus as well as in other areas of the brain (McGaugh, 2004).

The amygdala effectively supports explicit as well as implicit forms of memory.

There is evidence that suggests it is reasonable to conceive of the affect system as an early, primitive form of information processing and memory that now works both independently and in conjunction with the newer hippocampal memory system (LeDoux, 2002; MacLean, 1990). MacLean outlined the concept of the Triune Brain that describes the brain evolving by adding increasingly sophisticated systems for information processing, one layer on top of the next. Within such a conceptualization, the amygdala serves as the center for a mid-level information processing system. In some ways the amygdala operates in tandem with higher level, cortical information processing centers, but in many other ways it operates independently. Thus, while mood influences memory in the way Zajonc's research (1980) indicated, thereby triggering conscious memories consistent with the affect present at the time of recall (Dolan, 2000), emotion also operates quite independently of conscious processes (McGaugh, 2004). A pattern of sensory input can be viewed as triggering a specific emotion; the emotion can be viewed as distillation of the experience that then guides learning and action. Later in life, when a similar pattern of sensory input occurs for the individual, a similar emotion is triggered, similar information is called up, and a similar tendency toward action is expressed (Dolan, 2000).

Emotion as an information processing system tends to be experienced by the person as a "black box." That is, experience registered throughout the brain sends signals to the amygdala, and then an impulse to respond spits out the other end of the black box. Such information can be registered by the brain even when the person is not aware that the information has been presented (Dolan, 2000). To the conscious brain using declarative or narrative processing, it is difficult to explain how the brain arrived at the subsequent impulse. Too often, the impulse expressed in the emotion may run counter to the declarative, logical decision a person may make. As a result, emotions are experienced as out of control.

To the extent that being out of control is viewed as a sign of weakness, emotions are also viewed as signs of weakness. Considering emotions as a source of information can lead to a change in how a person reacts to emotions that are experienced. Rather than being something to be controlled and avoided, they become something to be respected as a source of information that can contribute to decisions about functioning. As conceived here, the frontal, cortical decision-making processes are viewed as more sophisticated and more flexible, but if the contribution of the emotional information processing system is denied, the more sophisticated processing system is missing some very important sources of information.

LeDoux (1996) has described the effects of varying levels of stress on the operations of the amygdala and the hippocampus. As stress levels rise from low to moderate, the production of noradrenaline stimulates both the amygdala and the hippocampus to work more effectively. At moderate stress levels it is therefore likely that conscious, explicit reactions to stimuli develop in synchrony with unconscious, direct, nonhippocampal reactions to stimuli. However, when stress is chronic, or when the stress reaction becomes extreme, as in the case of trauma, the higher noradenaline levels lead to reduced functioning in the hippocampus while facilitating processing with the amygdala. Length and branching of dendrites (neuronal extensions that receive input to the neuron) have been found to be reduced in the hippocampus subsequent to stress, and hippocampal cells have been found to die off in the presence of extremely high levels of stress. At the same time that explicit processing and narrative memory become ineffective, pairing of sensory stimuli with extremely powerful emotional reactions expressed in the amygdala becomes enhanced. The result of this combination of effects is that memories of powerful emotional events are likely to include effects on brain processing that are not part of the hippocampal system and therefore cannot be readily monitored consciously.

This conceptualization is different from the Freudian concept of repression, which delineates a failure in memory recall that avoids threatening material that would otherwise be available to conscious processing (LeDoux, 1996). Rather, the current model proposes that deficits in conscious recall of emotional material reflect the absence of neural connections that could allow explicit access to a traumatic memory. Flashbacks to trauma likely reflect the activation of connections between the amygdala and sensory and motor systems without activation of hippocampal systems. Recent neuroimaging research regarding flashbacks experienced by victims of Post Traumatic Stress Disorder provides strong evidence for a clear separation between autobiographical memory and flashbacks (Lanius *et al.*, 2004). Development of conscious awareness of overwhelming memories recorded in traumatic circumstances should be conceived as the development of new connections with a previously recorded implicit memory rather than as the removal of a blockage within connections that had previously been established. The operation of anxiety processes in the brain discussed in Chapter 6 are likely more congruent with the Freudian process of repression, but they do not preclude the presence the systems just described.

The concept of infantile amnesia discussed in Chapter 4 is particularly relevant to understanding early affect-laden memories. Long-term memory storage that includes hippocampal memory systems does not come "on line" until around the age of 3 or 4 years old because the neural substrates required for such memory have not yet developed (Squire *et al.*, 1993). A child's memories of emotional experiences during the first 3 to 4 years of life are therefore implicit memories, and it is unlikely an adult can have direct, conscious awareness of these events. Applying LeDoux's reasoning regarding early memories in general (1996), it seems likely that conscious awareness of early sensory memories and connected affect stored during these early years may sometimes be established as a newly constructed "memory of the memory". As with other early memories, it seems likely that early emotional memories will not be the same as memories of initial experiences stored using hippocampal systems later in life.

Affect, that is, emotion, clearly has a powerful influence on encoding as well as retrieval of information throughout the brain. As a central processor in the integration of emotion with information content, the amygdala serves memory by organizing input while also guiding recall of information. The amygdala has the potential to influence learning of nominally neutral information moving from input sensory systems through processing and out through verbal expression and behavior. The amygdala and emotional processing seem likely to serve a central role in the unfolding activation of neural networks. Within the context of psychotherapy, it therefore seems likely that attending to and influencing emotional activity can support understanding of a client's history while also facilitating positive change.

6

Anxiety

Anxiety is a final basic building block composing the brain foundation on which a conceptualization of psychotherapy interventions can be built. Gray and others have presented a model of anxiety as a warning system based on activity in specific areas of the hippocampus (the septo-hippocampal region) along with related areas in the prefrontal cortex and the amygdala (Blanchard *et al.*, 1993; Gray, 1982; Gray & McNaughton, 2003; McNaughton & Corr, 2004) (see Figure 6.1). They have described a monitoring system that can identify the similarity between current input and previous stimuli leading to punishment or nonreward. They have also suggested that there may be innate fear stimuli that serve as triggers for this system. As the organism is exposed to stimuli and experiences that lead to the firing of neuronal patterns previously tied to negative emotion, the warning system identifies the presence of this familiar negative pattern and triggers a response that includes increased arousal, increased attention to the environment, and behavioral inhibition.

Increased stress hormones have been found to interfere with retrieval of previous memories while simultaneously increasing the capacity to establish new memories (Roozendaal, 2002), so the triggering of the warning system may effectively "protect" the brain from remembering negative experiences

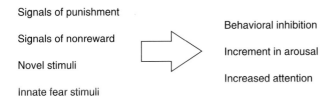

Anxiety: septal-hippocampal warning system

Figure 6.1 "Diagram of Gray's anxiety model (Gray, 1982)".

while facilitating learning new information in a potentially threatening setting. This suggests that anxiety blocks recollection while a person develops ways to reduce the immediate distress; this blocking results in a person avoiding memories previously associated with anxiety. Research on worry and brain activity has indicated that anxiety leads to diffuse brain arousal that may interfere with a person's capacity to process information effectively (Carter *et al.*, 1986). Concretely, if many parts of the brain are equally aroused it becomes harder to "hear" the message of any individual part of the brain. Studies of arousal and performance have long indicated that moderate levels of arousal may enhance functioning while high levels of arousal interfere with functioning (Yerkes & Dodson, 1908), a pattern that is consistent with the previously described disruption of hippocampal functioning in the presence of high stress (LeDoux, 1996).

This anxiety system appears to be congruent with the psychoanalytic concept of anxiety as a signal for beginning defensive action (Fenichel, 1945, pp. 132–4) and with cognitive behavioral conceptualizations (Barlow, 1988, p. 248). Anxiety is not viewed as a specific emotion; rather, it is a diffuse state of arousal associated with a variety of negative emotions. If a previously experienced stimulus has become paired with a negative emotional experience, then when new incoming stimulus patterns closely approximate the previous stimulus, the monitoring system proposed by Gray sounds the alarm. Incoming stimuli may include sensory input as well as proprioceptive (muscle related) and visceral (organ related) cues. Anxiety may disrupt brain functioning to such a degree that a person does not remember the pain previously associated with the stimulus. Behavioral inhibition contributes to avoiding continuing behaviors that can lead the organism closer to the source of the negative stimulus. Arousal may flood the brain, thereby interfering with the person recognizing the relevant previously encoded associations that led to the distress. Increased attention to the environment may limit internal awareness while also serving to prepare the person to identify external sources of danger if they emerge. Such responses may include defensive processes highlighted by Sigmund and Anna Freud (Fenichel, 1945).

Gray (1982) suggested that such a warning system also includes monitoring for identification of novel, unfamiliar patterns of stimulation. A brain pattern not previously associated with negative emotion may stimulate anxiety because it is new. In this model, the new pattern does not trigger anxiety because it has been previously associated with negative experiences. Rather, the new pattern triggers anxiety simply because it is not familiar. The model predicts that the anxiety reaction is the same whether the trigger is a novel stimulus or a familiar stimulus previously associated with negative events. It is therefore very likely that when someone experiences the anxiety associated with a novel stimulus, the person will experience the anxiety as indicating that something negative is happening in the environment.

Such a mechanism may account for difficulties some clients have in developing new, adaptive forms of behavior even though previous emotional conflicts appear to have been resolved. As the client begins to behave in adaptive but novel ways, anxiety is likely to be triggered and the patient will mistakenly infer that previous problems are still unresolved. Such an inference will lead the patient back into negative assessments of self and into maladaptive behaviors used in the past. The connection between novelty and anxiety also helps explain why people feel "at home" in maladaptive functioning and uncomfortable when functioning in new, more adaptive ways. It appears that the connection between novelty and anxiety can be so strong that remaining in abusive relationships is more bearable than taking steps to become more independent and therefore free of abuse.

Considering the novelty response in relation to the concept of neural network suggests an explanation for one source of interference with progress in psychotherapy. When a person is beginning to improve during the course of psychotherapy they should begin to behave in more adaptive ways. However, neural patterns associated with forms of adaptive functioning are likely to have relatively few links with other behavioral, emotional, or cognitive neural patterns in the brain. Therefore, when the adaptive behavior occurs, it is likely to fail to stimulate further neural patterns to fire. The result is likely to be an absence of brain activity. The client may decide to enter new social settings because the settings have been identified as healthy. However, once the client walks into the new setting he may not be able to come up with anything to say because there are no "next connections" in the brain. The client is then likely to experience anxiety, retreat in a panic, and view the experience as yet another sign of the permanence of inadequacy. The novelty of the new neural network combined with the lack of subsequent brain activity seems likely to trigger anxiety that interferes with personal progress in psychotherapy.

The inclusion of anxiety with the other elements of brain function that have been considered makes the picture of brain processing more complete. Information is taken in through various sensory systems and processed to the point of output by multiple discrete but integrated areas of the brain. Each experience is considered to consist of unique neural networks involving activity throughout the brain. Different memory systems process incoming information and contribute to neural networks in ways that influence the nature of these processes. Emotions influence processing, networks, and memory in ways that are obvious and subtle, conscious and unconscious. Finally, anxiety contributes to heightened consideration of the environment, rapid responding, and new learning while also having the potential to disrupt the retrieval of previously learned material. All of these elements of brain functioning operate simultaneously whereby the processing of initial sensory information is influenced by past learning, emotions, and anxiety that can be triggered almost immediately by incoming sensory information. Reciprocal signals moving back and forth between these different elements of brain processing shape a person's experiences through conscious as well as unconscious processes. Psychotherapy helps identify the nature of the processes and interactions that make up the client's functioning, and then it helps alter those processes and interactions to yield more successful living.

Before considering more completely the integration of brain activities just outlined, a final set of contributions to brain functioning needs to be elucidated. Thus far the elements of current functioning, for example, input–process–output elements, as well as integration of elements from the top to the bottom of the brain have been elaborated. It is now important to consider in more detail the developmental processes that influence the construction of the brain that supports previously considered elements of brain functioning. In the next two chapters, developmental processes will be outlined and themes and implications for functioning will be identified.

7

Processes of brain development

Basic elements of brain function previously outlined include the input–process–output neuropsychological conception of brain function, interactions between higher and lower levels of the brain, neural networks, explicit memory systems, implicit memory systems, affect systems, and anxiety systems. It is important to consider these elements interacting together as a finished product, but in order to understand the brain in psychotherapy it is crucial to understand how the end product was achieved.

The processes constituting brain development influence how different areas of the brain operate in psychotherapy for clients at various stages of maturation. The processes of brain development also influence how the brain encodes experiences during childhood and then recalls and applies these experiences during functioning in adulthood.

It is important to consider the influences of both genetics and experience on the development of brain function and personality. It is also important to understand the dual developmental processes of creating and then streamlining neural connections. Finally, it is important to recognize the influences of myelination on the integration and mature activation of brain systems. Consideration of these contributors to brain development can support a more complete understanding of how clients perceive events and respond to them in psychotherapy and throughout life.

Genetics

The genetic code with which each person is endowed at conception contains a range of potentials available to be realized (Gilliam *et al.*, 2000; Kramer, 2005). Some of the characteristics embedded in the code can be activated independent of events in the environment surrounding the organism. However, the expression of many characteristics embedded in the genetic code is modified by events in the environment, including the intrauterine environment (Kandel *et al.*, 2000b, chapters 52–8). Some potential characteristics embedded in the code may never emerge because of interactions between the genetic code and the environment. Some characteristics embedded in the genetic code may be blocked from appropriate development by the environment to the extent that brain functioning and related adaptive psychological functioning are severely disrupted or eliminated (Greenough *et al.*, 1987). Genes tell the neurons in the brain what to *try* to do. Interactions between genetics and the environment then determine what actually unfolds.

The processes underlying genetic influences are complex to the point of being overwhelming, and it is often difficult to identify direct connections between gene action and psychotherapy. However, recognition of some of the basic concepts related to genetic influences on brain function offers understanding of how psychological strengths and weaknesses develop and how they can be influenced.

Genetics influences the development of both psychopathology (Kramer, 2005; Shih *et al.*, 2004) and adaptive capacities (Greenough *et al.*, 1987). Examination of the prevalence of diagnosed mental disorders within families, among twins raised together, and among twins raised separately has provided evidence of the influence of inherited characteristics on the presence of major depressive disorder, bipolar disorder, panic, obsessive-compulsive disorder, and schizophrenia.

Recent developments in the areas of neural imaging and genetics have led to better understanding of how genes contribute to the development of psychopathology in offspring (Plomin & McGuffin, 2003). It appears that most psychiatric disorders are influenced by actions of multiple genes, and the tendency toward demonstration of symptoms of a disorder increases as the number of malfunctioning genes related to the disorder increases.

Genes contribute to phenotype, that is, observed characteristics and behavior, through processes of transcription, also called expression, and translation. Transcription is the process of sending a message from DNA in the gene to the cell regarding what function to undertake. Translation involves implementation of the specific chemical functions called for by the transcription from the gene. The presence of genes of a specific type as well as the absence of specific genes contribute to chemical processes within and between cells that eventually contribute to behavior identified as normal or abnormal. For example, it has been found that a specific genetic abnormality related to depression changes the production of a serotonin transporter within the cell. This change subsequently influences the reuptake from the synapse of serotonin, a neurotransmitter used in brain systems associated with depression. The result is an increased likelihood of symptoms of depression (Caspi *et al.*, 2003).

Genes are responsible for each step in a long series of chemical events extending from initial expression of the genetic message in the cell body of the neuron to final activity in the synapses that influences brain activity and behavior. Genes can disrupt this process at any point in this series of chemical events.

While it is clear that genes influence development of characteristics and behaviors, it is also becoming clear that "interplay" (Rutter, 2005) between genes and the environment strongly influences final development of phenotypic, that is, observed, behavior (Kramer, 2005). Studies described by Kramer have shown that changing the environment in which an animal is raised changes the behaviors the animal displays and also changes the production of neurotransmitters within the brain associated with demonstrated behavior. Similarly, Kramer discussed studies related to schizophrenia and to conduct disorder in humans that demonstrated patterns of interplay between genes and environment. When children of schizophrenic parents were adopted and raised in families subsequently rated as healthy or unhealthy, children raised in healthy families were much less likely to demonstrate symptoms of schizophrenia. When children with a specific genetic anomaly related to neurotransmitter function were compared to those without the anomaly, the combination of the anomaly and childhood maltreatment yielded significantly higher levels of conduct disorder and violent crime (Caspi *et al.*, 2003).

Studies of early development in humans and other mammals also indicate the presence of interplay between genetic and environmental influences in the development of specific areas of the brain and development of specific adaptive cognitive abilities. Examples of such interplays include the effects of negative social environment on children subjected to abuse and neglect (De Bellis, 2001) and the effects of specific patterns of optical stimulation on the development of the visual system in the cat (Hubel & Wiesel, 1970). The effects of optical stimulation on brain development are the basis for eye-patching interventions in the treatment of amblyopia in humans. Studies of sign language development in deaf clients suggest the presence of a similar critical underlying pattern of interplay between the developing brain and environmental experience during the development of language in humans (Newport, 1990).

Genetics definitely influences the cognitive, emotional, and behavioral functioning of clients by influencing brain activity within and between cells. Increasing understanding of the influence exerted by genes can lead to improved understanding of clients' functioning. But the evidence goes beyond adding mere understanding. Evidence that interaction with the environment influences whether and how genes influence behavior strongly indicates that medical and social interventions, including psychotherapy, can influence brain activity toward adaptive functioning. This appears to be the case even when an underlying genetic predisposition is inclined toward maladaptive functioning (Kramer, 2005).

The genetic code, established at the time of conception, influences all aspects of brain function throughout life. The code, in interplay with the environment, guides the unfolding of all processes of brain development. Processes of brain development important to consider are neuron migration, arborization, synaptogenesis, pruning, and myelination. Migration is the process of neurons moving to the right location in the brain. Arborization is the process of extending dendrites and axons, the branches of the neurons, toward the appropriate neurons in other parts of the brain. Synaptogenesis is the development of connections between one neuron and another. Pruning involves the elimination of some neurons and neuronal connections in order to increase the efficiency of other connections and of the brain as a whole. Myelination is the process of insulating established axons and dendrites, thereby increasing the speed of signal transmission in neurons and making brain function more efficient.

Migration

Neurons are produced during early gestation in the neural tube and then later in the ventricles in the central areas of the brain (Marin & Rubenstein, 2003). Once produced, the neurons migrate to their genetically coded appropriate positions in the brain. During migration, cells move from the ventricles where they are generated to layers closer to the surface of the forming brain.

In the end the cortex is composed of six layers of neurons arranged in columns. The earliest neurons produced compose the layer of the cortex nearest to the center. Subsequent layers are added one on top of the next over the course of gestation. Neurons destined for each subsequent layer must pass through the layers that have already been established in order to reach their appropriate locations.

The various chemical processes that guide migration are vulnerable to disruption during gestation (Cicchetti & Cannon, 1999). Genetic anomalies in mice demonstrate specific problems with migration that subsequently disrupt brain organization and behavior. It has been established that substance abuse during migration results in severe subsequent disruption of a person's brain functioning with impairments in processes such as focusing attention, managing affect, managing arousal, and integrating information (Guerri, 1998). There is also evidence that, when the mother experiences depression, anxiety, or stress, the chemical byproducts of these experiences enter the child's forming brain and influence subsequent development (Cicchetti & Cannon, 1999; Hayashi et al., 1998).

When a neuron fails to migrate to the correct location, several subsequent processes can be disrupted (Purves & Lichtman, 1985). The neuron will not be in the right location to receive axons of other neurons that grow toward a genetically defined specific location to connect with the neuron. The neuron will not be in the right location from which to extend axons to appropriate receptor neurons. And the neuron may either receive axons from or extend axons to inappropriate neurons so that signals intended to facilitate one type of brain response instead facilitate another, thereby causing disrupted mental processing. Researchers studying schizophrenia have hypothesized that schizophrenia is strongly influenced by disturbed cell migration in the hippocampal region (Kotrla *et al.*, 1997) and other areas (Arnold, 1999). The typical onset of schizophrenia during the period of late adolescence is accounted for by the fact that in the course of development the neurons that have migrated inappropriately during gestation do not typically become integrated into cognitive functioning until late adolescence. The result is that a gestational disturbance of migration results in a change that does not become evident for 20 years.

Arborization and synaptogenesis

During gestation and during the first 2 years of life massive numbers of new connections between neurons are formed. Arborization is one of the primary processes supporting the development of these connections (Arnold, 1999; Kandel *et al.*, 2000b; Purves & Lichtman, 1985). Axons grow from one neuron toward genetically predetermined locations in other parts of the brain, sometimes traveling to the far side of the brain, establishing connections throughout the brain. Simultaneously, dendrites branch out to receive other neurons offering input.

At the same time that arborization is occurring, the creation of new synapses, that is, synaptogenesis, is supported by mutual activity in connected cells. When a neuron fires, thereby sending a signal to a receiving neuron, and the receiving neuron also fires, the activity in the receiving neuron triggers the production of chemical products that encourage the development of new synapses connecting the two neurons and that help strengthen and maintain synapses that have already been established (Kandel *et al.*, 2000b; Purves & Lichtman, 1985). These chemicals also support the continuing survival of the neurons. Neuronal activity promotes the establishment of stronger connections between neurons by encouraging more dendritic branching, encouraging creation of more synapses, and increasing the strength of individual synapses. These processes result in the establishment of more and stronger connections between the simultaneously active neurons.

Whereas the chemical milieu seems to be a primary influence on the generation and initial migration of neurons, during arborization and synaptogenesis it appears that neuronal activity becomes a more prominent influence on the establishment of connections between neurons. Activity in target-connecting neurons leads to the production of chemical agents such as Nerve Growth Factor that support new arborization, creation of synapses, and maintenance of connections that have already been made (Arnold, 1999; Kandel et al., 2000b; Purves & Lichtman, 1985). Studies have shown that the brain cortices of animals raised in highly stimulating environments are heavier (Bennett et al., 1964; Greenough et al., 1987) and have more synapses than the brains of animals raised in non-stimulating environments. Because it appears that early experiences substantially influence arborization and synaptogenesis, it can be said that early experiences influence the "wiring" that is laid down in the brain during the early years. Thus, early childhood learning is different from adult learning in that adult learning can be viewed as influencing how already established wiring fires, but not as influencing so strongly the shape of the wiring. While this difference between the natures of childhood and adult learning seems to be relatively accurate, it should also be noted that studies of learning in adults suggest that some elements of the wiring process remain open to change through experience even though the relative extent of such change is lower in adulthood than in childhood (Chklovskii et al., 2004; Mitchell et al., 2004; Reuter-Lorenz, 2002).

Pruning

The first 2–4 years of brain development are characterized by a proliferation in interneuronal connections. After 2 years of age the process of pruning begins to predominate. The massive numbers of synapses established during the first years of life begin to die off in a process of cutthroat competition. Chugani and Chugani (1997) studied glucose metabolism, which is associated with maintenance of synapses, and the data clearly outlined the impact of pruning over the course of childhood and adolescence (see Figure 7.1). It appears that synapses and neurons that are not used regularly wither away, leaving behind the synapses and neurons that are most active. It appears that the receptor neurons only produce a limited amount of the chemicals needed to maintain synaptic connections, and synapses that are not regularly used do not receive these chemicals (Johnston, 2004; Kandel et al., 2000b; Purves & Lichtman, 1985). The process is a way for the brain to adapt itself to the environment in which it finds itself. The synapses and neurons regularly stimulated by the environment are the ones likely to be maintained. The end result is a brain

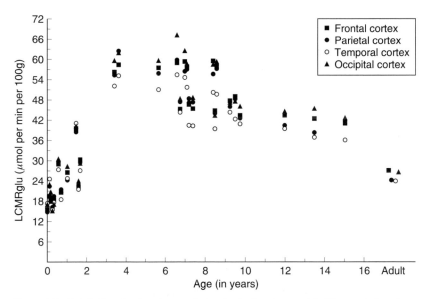

Figure 7.1 Metabolic rates for glucose during brain development (with permission, from Chugani & Chugani, 1997).

that works much more quickly and efficiently in processing information (Casey *et al.*, 2000).

It appears that the same interactions between the brain and the environment that lead to the initial establishment and maintenance of synapses help shape the subsequent pruning: "Use it or lose it!" Regular mutual firing of neurons helps generate the chemicals that maintain a synapse, while lack of regular mutual firing leads to the synapse's demise. The child's consistent interactions with people, the regular repetition of behaviors, and repeated rehearsal of emotions paired with events shape the brain and its subsequent ability to process information and relationships.

Myelination

The final major process of brain development that needs to be considered is myelination. This is the process whereby glial cells wrap axons of neurons in an insulating sheath that facilitates a marked increase in speed of transmission of electrical impulses along the length of the axon. Various areas of the brain have been found to typically complete myelination at different ages (see Figure 7.2), with the cross modal integration areas and the frontal lobes being the last to become myelinated (Yakolev & Lecours, 1967).

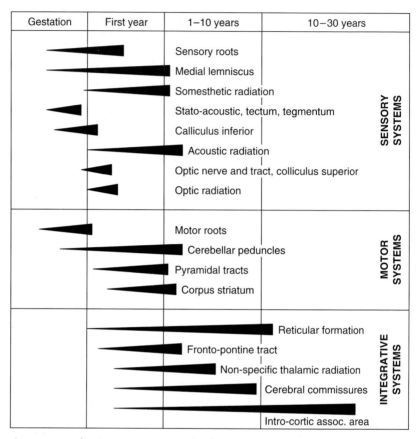

Gestation	First year	1–10 years	10–30 years

Sensory roots
Medial lemniscus
Somesthetic radiation
Stato-acoustic, tectum, tegmentum
Calliculus inferior
Acoustic radiation
Optic nerve and tract, colliculus superior
Optic radiation

SENSORY SYSTEMS

Motor roots
Cerebellar peduncles
Pyramidal tracts
Corpus striatum

MOTOR SYSTEMS

Reticular formation
Fronto-pontine tract
Non-specific thalamic radiation
Cerebral commissures
Intro-cortic assoc. area

INTEGRATIVE SYSTEMS

Figure 7.2 Myelination patterns across development (with permission, adapted from Yakolev & Lecours, 1967).

Myelination is particularly important for cross-modal integration of information because long axons are required to bring in information from distant areas of the brain. If long axons are operating slowly, integration is impaired (Kandel *et al.*, 2000b). As the myelination process is completed in the frontal lobes, decision making and "stop and think" impulse control procedures become active and available for helping a person manage thought, emotion, and action (Durston *et al.*, 2001; Nagy *et al.*, 2004). Late myelination is one of the reasons that long-term thinking and planfulness do not become well developed before adolescence. This late completion of the wiring in of the frontal lobes offers some hope to those working with impulsive children in that even though impulsivity has not been managed by less mature mechanisms earlier in development, it may be possible for alternate mechanisms in the frontal lobes to provide such self-control.

This final wave of development can be considered to have arrived a moment too late. That is, the hormonal tide of puberty appears to typically arrive somewhat before the final keys to impulse control and decision making are in place; hence, the somewhat rocky period known as early adolescence (ages 11–13 years). Hormones appear to stimulate subcortical systems that contribute to increases in acting out of emotion (Durston *et al.*, 2001). As discussed earlier, influences in the brain flow from the lower brain systems toward the top as well as from the top to the bottom (Derryberry & Tucker, 1992). Increases in emotionality can therefore be expected to both directly and indirectly influence thought and action mediated by higher cortical processing. The typical adolescent progression from overly dramatic to considered and planful seems likely to mirror the increasing influence of frontal executive systems in the overall working of the brain.

The processes described in this chapter tend to unfold during development following the sequence outlined. However, there is much overlap in the periods during which these processes are active. There are also indications that these processes proceed at varying rates in different parts of the maturing brain (Casey *et al.*, 2000), and may continue to varying degrees throughout life. Myelination of long axons supporting complex integration is a critical process during adolescence and early development, but it also occurs as early as gestation (Durston *et al.*, 2001). There are indications of ongoing generation of specific types of new cells in the hippocampus during adulthood (Schmidt-Hieber *et al.*, 2004), and there are signs that some types of cells continue to migrate during adulthood (Marin & Rubenstein, 2003). Synaptogenesis, arborization, and pruning all appear to continue throughout adulthood, albeit at lower rates than during the explosive unfolding of early developmental years (Arnold, 1999). The influences each of these processes has on brain activity can thus extend to periods other than those emphasized in the current description of developmental processes.

There are a number of implications and patterns inherent in the unfolding developmental processes just described. Chapter 8 identifies some of these patterns and implications explicitly and summarizes the relationships between developmental processes and the overall framework of brain functioning presented in chapters 2 through 6.

8

Themes of brain development

In order to understand psychological functioning in children as well as in adults it is important to understand how the processes unfolding during brain development influence psychological functioning over the course of development. Until recently, differences between the workings of children's brains and adults' brains were poorly recognized (if they were acknowledged at all). Medieval painters captured the issue on canvas: Madonna and Child paintings in the fifteenth century often presented Mary holding a tiny mature adult man in her lap rather than an infant; the image of the infant was treated as if the child was a miniature adult.

It is now recognized that a child's brain functions much differently than does an adult's brain, but often the extent and nature of the differences between the adult's brain and the child's brain are not fully appreciated. Adequate appreciation should include recognition that children's brains absorb, perceive, process, and respond to experiences in ways that are different from the processing in adult's brains. Adequate appreciation of differences should also include understanding that much of the information held in the mature, adult brain was taken in and integrated when the brain was much less developed and, as a result, much of the information on which the adult brain relies for processing current experiences is immature in structure and activity.

With regard to psychotherapy, interventions with a child's brain call for different approaches than interventions with an adult's brain. This is due to the availability of different capacities and processes. Intervening with an adult regarding early childhood experiences requires that therapist and client recognize that memories and emotional reactions are often based on immature brain functioning despite the adult client's wish to respond in a mature, adaptive fashion.

A profound implication of the rapidly developing nature of the child's brain is that many connections in the brain are not yet established and as a result the processes associated with those connections are not available either.

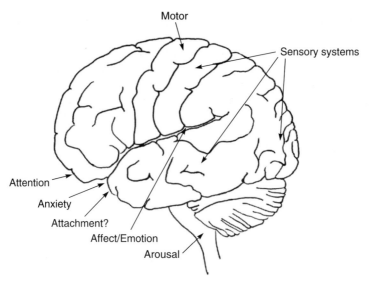

Figure 8.1 Brain with functions schematically represented without integration processes.

Observing Figure 8.1, it is striking what is available and what is not. During the first years of a child's life various areas of the brain move from being very inactive to being very active. Areas of the brain related to sensation, motor activity, emotion, attachment, and anxiety tend to be available early in development, and behavioral and cognitive skills that rely on these areas develop more quickly. Frontal lobe decision-making and major integration areas present in Figure 1.1 are absent in Figure 8.1, and because skills related to these areas are not available to the child, assessment and planning are much weaker early in life than they will be as the child moves toward adulthood (see Teeter & Semrud-Clikeman, 1997, chapter 2).

Particular characteristics of brain development are useful to consider. Brain systems underlying implicit memory processes, explicit memory processes, affect, and anxiety all unfold during the course of development. During development the nature and influence of memory, emotion, and anxiety all shift, and the influence each of these elements of brain functioning has on learning and personality development changes as well. Different areas of the brain develop at different rates and, as a result, different capacities become available for inclusion in psychological functioning at different times. Furthermore, different areas of the brain reach the end of the period of heightened plasticity (that is, capacity to change and develop) at different times. When an area of the brain reaches the end of heightened plasticity, high level capacities for specific types of learning and development come to an end as well.

As the various areas of the brain develop, activity in one area of the brain can strongly influence development and activity in other areas of the brain. Finally, the person's experiences can strongly influence brain development occurring at the time of the experience, resulting in immediate as well as delayed consequences. Elaboration of each of these processes or interactions is important for adequate understanding of the influences of development on psychological functioning.

Implicit memory systems

A notable characteristic of childhood memory and learning is that processes related to implicit memory rather than explicit, hippocampal memory form the basis of learning during the earliest years. People typically have "childhood amnesia" for events experienced during the first several years of life (Siegel, 1999). Short periods of awareness appear to emerge to some degree several months after birth, suggesting that hippocampal integration is somewhat active, but the processes required for long-term storage of such events are limited or non-existent.

By default, implicit memory processes are the bedrock of learning during the first several years of development. Direct neuronal connections and connections in primary association areas integrating sensation, arousal, affect, and motor systems are the primary bases for learning. Learning is founded on repeated paired activation of neurons in these various systems rather than on processes such as insight and conscious understanding based on hippocampal and frontal lobe functioning. Associations are learned slowly through repetition and will be resistant to change. Because these connections between affect, experience, and behavior are being established without inclusion of long-term, hippocampal memory systems, it may never be possible to retrieve these memories and include them in the conscious narrative history maintained by the person.

Informal observation and formal research (Stern, 1985) have provided powerful evidence that even in the absence of long-term declarative or explicit memory, important learning occurs during the early years. Infants quickly learn to respond differentially to the mother's scent. Development of language and motor skills provides the most obvious evidence of learning during the first several years of life, but there is also strong evidence that learning pairing emotions with events is occurring as well. Such basic learning appears to be occurring at birth if not before. It is likely that early experiences such as crying in response to the discomfort of a dirty diaper being followed by the face of Father and a changed dry diaper contribute to the development of positive emotional reactions to the face of Father as well as to a deeply held, growing pattern of self-efficacy on the part of the child.

Research on early learning has shown that in early years many more repetitions of an event are required for learning to occur than are required in later years, but occur it does (Bauer, 2004). Implied is the need for high levels of consistency and repetition in the child's environment if connections are to be made and stabilized.

Not only does learning of associations occur because of repetition, but the connections needed for future learning are also established. Arborization, synaptogenesis, and pruning all suggest the importance of such consistency and repetition; if consistent patterns of experience do not occur, the brain will not establish the neural connections required for later processing, or will not maintain these connections if they have been established. When consistency is lacking in the childhood environment, the potential for future learning is diminished. The genetic potential thus fails to unfold due to the lack of consistent patterns in the child's environment.

Affect

Emotional responses learned by the brain during the early, "implicit memory" period will continue to affect perception, mood, and behavior in ways that may seem unreasonable and out of control to the adult brain dealing with these responses years later. This is particularly likely to be true if the experiences of the first several years are at odds with memories from later years. A significant period of poor caretaking during the first 2 years of life may leave emotional traces that never make sense to the individual if the patterns of parenting have become more supportive since that time.

MacLean (1990) has conceptualized the limbic system as a primitive learning system, and it appears that this system is active before long-term declarative memory is active. As a result, repeated pairing of specific emotions with specific external sensations will result in a learned emotional response to the sensory stimulus. If Mother regularly soothes the distressed child effectively, the child is likely to develop a positive emotional response to the image of Mother. If mothering interventions are inconsistent, the establishment of such a positive emotional bond is less likely; in fact, such an unpredictable pattern may contribute to a generally disorganized quality of cognitive processing. Finally, if Mother is angry and irritable in her responses to any indication of distress in the child, the child is likely to develop a strongly negative emotional response to the image of Mother, with subsequent generalization of disrupted relatedness throughout life. All relationships are then likely to be experienced with anxiety and distress even if conscious assessment of adult relationships cannot discern the bases for such reactions.

Anxiety

The interaction between affect and anxiety is important to remember when considering early childhood learning since the interaction can unfold with few signs that are obvious to the adults involved. The anxiety model proposed by Gray suggests that if a child regularly experiences pain or discomfort as a result of an adult's interactions with the child, the child will begin to develop an anxiety response associated with sensations that are part of the experience of that adult, such as seeing the adult's face or hearing the adult's voice. The child may develop a similar anxiety reaction in response to proprioceptive distress; that is, if the child is inconsistently soothed when hungry, the anxiety system may be triggered by the sensation of hunger itself. However, if the child is consistently soothed when hungry, the beginning pangs of hunger may not develop into a trigger for the onset of anxiety. Finally, if soothing and pain are both very unpredictable, the child may develop little capacity to predict or control the environment, and a chronic state of vigilance can develop that is overly effortful and draining for the person as a child and as an adult. Because early childhood learning tends to be procedural rather than declarative in nature, it is possible that none of the patterns just described would be consciously available to the person to be recognized even though the pattern has a strong influence on the functioning of the person.

The non-declarative but powerful nature of learning in early childhood has an important implication for adults working with or raising small children. Adults are tempted to disregard their interactions with the child during the early years because the influence of early interactions is not immediately obvious and because the adult's own conscious memory of similar early childhood events is nonexistent. Adults are therefore at risk to engage in patterns of behavior that leave negative emotional reactions to adults and relationships in the child's brain. If Father chooses to work long hours during the child's early years with the expectation that the bond will be available to be established later, Father may be sadly surprised by the teenage child's lack of response.

The procedural nature of early learning suggests that once learned, implicit memory patterns will be very resistant to change. The implication is that even though someone might later become aware of the interpersonal interaction patterns that led to the development of a specific emotional reaction early in life, simple insight will not be likely to undo the pairing thus established.

Instead, multiple rehearsals of a competing interpersonal pattern would be required in order for habituation to occur. Even then, the implication of the hard wiring nature of early learning is that neural connections that support the recurrence of the maladaptive emotional reaction are likely to remain, and so the person is likely to remain vulnerable to recurrence of the emotional reaction pattern even though the issue was resolved earlier.

Explicit memory

Long-term memory processes associated with declarative learning seem to become actively established between the ages of 2 and 4 years old (Bauer, 2004). The hippocampus as an integration area becomes progressively more active as a means of managing experiences. Encoding of new information as well as reprocessing of old become progressively more influenced by declarative memory processes including insight, context, and planfulness (LeDoux, 1996).

Cross modal integration centers in the parietal and temporal areas of the brain also become more active, supporting higher levels of conceptualization and increased capacity for organizing and analyzing information. The parietal areas develop into centers in which language is integrated with vision, sound, touch, action, and affect. Language thus becomes a progressively more powerful tool for managing information (Durston *et al.*, 2001).

Developmental patterns

Consideration of each of several patterns of development that occur in various areas of the brain can contribute to a richer understanding of psychological development in children, adolescents, and adults. Different regions of the brain become active at different stages of development, influencing the capacities available for learning and taking action. Different regions of the brain reach a point at which capacity to change becomes markedly reduced, resulting in subsequent unavailability for new development. Activity and development in one area of the brain can substantially increase or impede development in other areas of the brain. Finally, experiences can profoundly influence the way in which specific areas of the brain develop, thereby markedly altering capacity for future functioning.

Different brain systems come on line at different times (Greenough & Black, 1992; Greenough *et al.*, 1987; Knudsen, 2004). That is, there are "sensitive periods", "critical periods", or "developmental windows" during which specific areas of the brain are most available to developing while interacting with the environment. The developing child will not have certain behavioral capacities available until the underlying neural mechanisms are in place. For example, if the neural underpinnings of toilet training are not in place at the age of 2 years old when common social practice would indicate, the parents will be pressuring the child to do the impossible if they emphasize bowel or bladder control. The child is likely to feel overwhelmed and to experience himself as inadequate. The risk is high that the child will become defiant with regard to toilet training in particular, a pattern that may initiate the development of a neural network supporting oppositionality as a way to gain control in life. Similarly, if eager parents press the child to begin to write before the necessary underlying neural structures have developed adequately, it is possible that writing will become associated with anxiety and feelings of incompetence that can interfere with future progress in this area. The potential benefits of early repetitive firing in relevant synapses will be lost in the face of the negative effects of anxiety and an avoidant neural network pattern.

While some neural systems required for expression of certain behaviors do not come on line until a certain point, the periods of optimum growth for some other brain systems come to a close by certain ages (Greenough & Black, 1992; Greenough et al., 1987; Knudsen, 2004). "Windows of development" open and close during the earliest years as well as during later development. This appears to be true for the brain in general in that the first 25 years of life are characterized by maximum malleability overall. However, some areas of the brain appear to be more influenced by the opening and closing of developmental windows than are others (Bennett et al., 1964).

There are indications that attachment centers in humans, mimicking the imprinting of some lower animals, may become less available to influence after the first several years of life, and that if repetitions of loving touch have not occurred by that time, the nature of the person's bonds with those with whom the person is closest will be permanently limited (Schore, 1994). Studies of children who experienced neglect by parenting figures indicate that specific areas of the brain are underdeveloped (Teicher et el., 2004). Infants who have experienced emotional and tactile deprivation display aberrant production of stress hormones (Glaser, 2000), and children with similar backgrounds have been found to have a higher rate of attachment problems after adoption (O'Connor et al., 2003). If a child languishes in the crib while the depressed mother watches television during the first 2 years of the child's life, it is likely that attachment will not occur effectively and may never have the same automatic quality in subsequent relationships. Similarly, if language has not developed within the first 10–12 years of life, the neural connections related to language functioning appear to become solidified and less amenable to influence. Language fluency is then likely to be permanently impaired (Newport, 1990).

Activity in one brain system can influence the development of other systems (Knudsen, 2004). Problems with attention can reduce a child's capacity to focus long enough on a series of events to begin to develop understanding of those events. Conceptually, if the sensory, motor, and integration neurons related to those events do not fire repeatedly together because poor attention prevents the child from recognizing the unfolding series of events, it is surmised that subsequent permanent wiring in those sensory, motor, and integration systems will be limited. Disruptive firing of affect neurons as a result of underlying mood or seizure disorders can similarly be predicted to disrupt development of neuronal integration necessary for processing relationships in the environment. Associations between neurons are then likely to be based on internally generated cues and, as a result, the brain's capacity to interact with the environment in adaptive ways is reduced.

The implications of the disruptive impact of attention problems or mood disorders suggest early rather than late intervention, even when the immediate impact of the attention problem is relatively benign. That is, if intervention for attention problems is delayed because the young child is small and therefore easily controllable, important opportunities for brain development may be missed due to prolonged lack of focus and inconsistent activation of neuron pairs related to accurate perception of and reaction to events in the environment.

Because it appears that early experiences substantially influence arborization, synaptogenesis, and pruning, it can be said that early experiences affect the wiring that is installed in the brain during the early years. Thus, early childhood learning is different from adult learning in that adult learning can be viewed as influencing how already established wiring fires, but not as influencing so strongly the shape of the wiring.

Interactions with caregivers appear to strongly influence the development of brain systems related to attachment, affect regulation, and general cognitive processing (Kinniburgh et al., 2005; Schore, 1994). As a result, not only do early experiences leave implicit memory traces that affect subsequent interactions with the environment, they also shape the structure of the brain in ways that alter the individual's capacity to process information and relationships.

Building of neuronal connections followed by planned pruning is a primary means whereby the environment leaves its indelible mark on the person's character (Greenough et al., 1987). Early experiences power-fully shape permanent wiring. The brain is thus molded to match the environment around it and to optimize its effectiveness within that environment. Observing the patterns of thought, emotion, and behavior that emerge during therapy reveals the tell-tale residuals of early experience, and can guide the therapist toward better understanding of how the person came to be and how they are most likely to be influenced toward adaptive change.

The effects of maltreatment and abuse during the early developmental years offer a graphic example of the potential for experience to affect brain development. Adults diagnosed with Post Traumatic Stress Disorder related to childhood abuse have been found to have reduced volume and activity of brain areas related to attention focusing, emotional processing, autobiographical working memory, and language (Ford, 2005). Evidence has been found for damage to the hippocampi as a consequence of stress and abuse in animals and humans during early childhood (Andersen & Teicher, 2004; De Bellis, 2001). There are some signs that very early intervention in the form of positive parenting may attenuate the negative effects of early abuse (Andersen & Teicher, 2004), but it appears most likely that physiological effects of early abuse will affect cognitive and emotional processing throughout the lifespan.

Identification of the profound effects of early experiences on childhood brain development combined with identification of processes such as the closing of developmental windows suggests limitations of the individual's potential to change as an adult. Even though the view that immature brains are more available to change than adult brains seems to be relatively accurate, it should also be noted that studies of learning in adults are beginning to suggest that some elements of the wiring remain open to change through experience even though the relative extent of such change is lower in adulthood than in childhood (Cicchetti & Cannon, 1999).

During late adolescence and early adulthood the final pieces of the brain structure and function "puzzle" fall in to place. Pruning streamlines brain activity, making it more efficient, and myelination supports the addition of executive decision-making and self-control mechanisms to declarative and procedural memory systems, neural networks, affective connections, and anxiety. The brain with all its functions as depicted in Figure 1.1 has emerged.

9

Basic concepts: summary and integration

Before exploring the clinical implications of brain systems and processes described in previous chapters it is worthwhile to summarize the ideas that have been presented thus far and organize these ideas within a framework that can guide conceptualization and intuition. Such an organizational framework can support a concrete and somewhat simplified view of brain functioning that can facilitate the application of neuroscience knowledge to psychotherapy intervention.

Information can be viewed as entering the brain through any of a number of sensory avenues to be integrated in multiple parallel centers, recombined in novel ways, and expressed through a variety of output pathways. Paths of influence within the brain flow from lower arousal mechanisms, up to mid-brain affect and integration systems, then to the higher cortex, and back again, in a continuous reciprocal flow. Connections can be direct as well as mediated by intervening connections as information flows up and down the brain. Each thought, experience, or action can be conceived as based on an underlying neural network composed of neurons from disparate parts of the brain, and each network can be understood to have connections with other networks through the sharing of neurons that compose each network. Implicit, procedural memory processes support emotional and non-emotional learning within and outside the awareness of the individual, while explicit, declarative memory systems relying on the hippocampus and associated frontal cortex systems support complex integration and rapid analysis of information in the brain. Affect systems centered in the amygdala can be viewed as primitive processing centers receiving sensory information and influencing thought and action in ways that are often beneath the awareness of the individual; however, activity in the amygdala can also be consciously experienced as emotions that seem out of control and frighteningly powerful. Anxiety, conceived as mediated by the septo-hippocampal warning system, develops as an alarm for the triggering of preparedness for adaptive action that can include maladaptive defensive procedures as well as adaptive arousal.

Brain development unfolds in ways that permanently shape all of the neural connections mediating the processes just described. Understanding brain development contributes to understanding how brain structures support function at any given point in the course of development. At the same time, understanding brain development offers insights into why the client's adult brain is currently structured as it is and why it functions as it does. On the one hand, concepts regarding brain function can be understood in light of developmental influences; on the other hand, these concepts can also contribute to an overall framework that can guide conceptualization of the adult brain during psychotherapy.

The various individual elements described thus far can be conceived as a collection of processes constituting an individual person's unique functioning. Each person takes in information through various sensory modalities and processes the information at progressively more complex levels. Eventually this processing leads to a variety of potential response alternatives that is unique for each person. Different individuals have differing strengths and weaknesses in their intake, processing, and output systems, and understanding these differences is useful in developing psychotherapy interventions.

The input–process–output flow for each person can be viewed as an array of neural networks that is different from the arrays that develop for any other person. For a given person, any given neuron can be included in a variety of neural network patterns, with the pattern rather than the individual neuron accounting for the specific neural representation of the experience. Neurons in one pattern are shared with other patterns, and this sharing can result in one pattern triggering the firing of another pattern with which it shares neurons. Associations between patterns likely develop as a result of these interconnections. Each neural network and each array of neural networks is derived from interplay between the person's genetic endowment and life experiences. During psychotherapy, attending to and following patterns of connection within and between neural networks guides identification of each client's problems and development of individualized resolutions.

Emotions appear to be extremely effective in triggering activity in neural network patterns, so a pattern that includes a given emotion is likely to trigger other patterns that include the same emotion. In this way, emotions help record unique associations between related stimuli that have developed for a person. Emotions also help connect current experiences with past experiences in ways that are different for each individual, and attending to the way emotions of the moment trigger recall of past experiences guides understanding of the client. Furthermore, working to actively manage emotions can help shifts in therapy occur, with specific patterns of emotional connection and avenues for change varying from person to person.

The input–process–output flow and activity within and between neural networks operate within explicit and implicit memory systems in ways that vary from person to person. Genetics and experience interact to offer a unique pattern of memory capabilities. Hippocampal memory systems including multiple frontal connections appear to underlie conscious, narrative, explicit memory that a person can recall with awareness. Levels of effectiveness of these systems vary widely from person to person, so some people may be able to readily experience and influence their own brain functioning in conscious and intentional ways, while other people may not be able to effectively use these memory systems. Hippocampal memory systems are especially vulnerable to environmental insults ranging from hypoxia to stress to abuse, so recognizing a person's declarative memory capacities can guide understanding of a person's past, identification of the person's current strengths, and intervention with the person during psychotherapy.

There are multiple nonhippocampal memory systems, with each type of memory using different areas of the brain. Nonhippocampal systems support processes that strongly effect behavior and intuition but are typically not conscious. As with other aspects of brain processing, each person has an individual pattern of strengths and weaknesses in these various systems. For example, one person may be more strongly influenced by implicit visual systems while another may be more influenced by implicit auditory systems. Incorporation, processing, and expression of nonhippo-campal implicit memory activities are likely to occur outside a person's awareness, but these activities are nonetheless observable, accessible to external influence, and unique.

Frequently explicit and implicit memory systems work in a simultaneous and integrated fashion, but they can also operate independently. The patterns of interaction between implicit and explicit processes will vary across individuals. Within each individual, the availability of specific types of experience and information to implicit and explicit processing is also likely to vary. Some people may be able to intentionally and consciously consider emotions tied to various experiences and feelings, while other people may be affected by emotions primarily through implicit, unconscious channels.

Of particular importance is the fact that emotion can be included in neural network patterns that have no connection with hippocampal memory systems. Emotions can therefore influence cognitive functioning without a person having any awareness of this processing. Furthermore, some people may have available neural systems for verbal processing that

The Big Picture

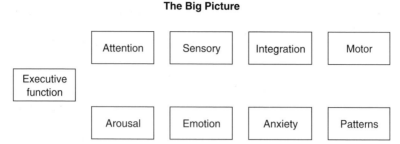

Figure 9.1 The "Big Picture": primary elements of the neuroscience in psychotherapy model.

can be applied to processing emotions, while other people who function well in many ways may not have substantial access to such verbal processing.

Finally, anxiety can be conceived as an individualized warning system that identifies the imminent arrival of a negative stimulus. While most individuals have an anxiety system that responds to potentially dangerous situations, genetics and especially experience result in each person having a unique pattern of anxiety activation and intensity. Anxiety responses can prepare a person to deal with a threatening situation, but they can also interfere with awareness of internal neural patterns through over-activity in the brain and through the generation of defensive responses designed to reduce anxiety. These defensive responses are likely to interfere with the development of adaptive responses.

Furthermore, an anxiety response can be triggered by novel experiences. In patterns unique to each individual, novelty-based anxiety can interact with the absence of connections between an unfamiliar, novel adaptive neural network and other neural networks associated with behavior, affect, and thought; this interaction can lead to regression in functioning even though progress is being made in therapy.

The elements of brain functioning can be integrated into a conceptual "Big Picture" presented in Figure 9.1. This figure lays out the "pieces and steps" elements of the input–process–output model in the top row along with the "combinations" elements of the neural network model in the bottom row. The box representing executive functioning is located to the middle left to emphasize its role in guiding general brain functioning through activation and inhibition, and to highlight its role in coordinating cognitive processing with arousal, emotional, and anxiety states. The "patterns" element in the bottom row refers to specific patterns of experience in a person's life that regularly influence the ways a person perceives situations and responds in specific settings or specific types of interactions.

The figure could have been drawn with arrows representing direction of influence from each box in the figure to every other box, thereby representing the complex reciprocal interconnections between the many areas of the brain active during processing. However, the outcome of including such arrows would be a meaningless cloud of vectors. Each element has multiple connections with each other area, and there is feedback between all connected elements. Even in the step-wise connections represented in the top half of the diagram, there are feed-forward and feed-back loops demonstrating that any one part of the brain influences the firing of any other part of the brain.

Each experience consists of all the individual elements being active to one degree or another. "Snapshots" of experience, for example, psychological assessment results or moments in psychotherapy, can be characterized as being influenced by higher levels of activity in some elements of the model and by less activity in others.

Breakdowns in functioning, whether through lack of activity in an element or over-activity in an element, can be conceived as occurring within specific elements, and the subsequent disruption in the overall system can be characterized by identifying the specific influences the disrupting element has on other elements. For example, disruption in arousal can lead to breakdowns throughout the system. The eighth-grade athlete who has problems with managing arousal may be so excited about playing in the upcoming soccer game that the focusing elements of attention are "drowned out" by the over-excitation of all elements of the input–process–output system; he cannot pay attention in class on the day of the game, so he cannot integrate new information being taught. At the same time, global arousal can stimulate his motor system to the point that minimal excitation from peers in the lunchroom results in the student beginning to shove others in a playful but aggressive way that leads to disciplinary action including not being allowed to participate in the game that was exciting him in the first place.

Successful functioning can similarly be characterized in terms of the relative contributions of various elements to the specific experience. Success in academic work may be due to high activity levels in executive and attention systems accompanied by only average capacity to process information and activate relevant patterns of thought. In such a situation, the student succeeds because the student is able to focus intently and generate long periods of effort (see Figure 9.2). Alternatively, a student might be highly distractible while having strong ability to process facts and carry out decision-making and reasoning tasks. With this alternative pattern

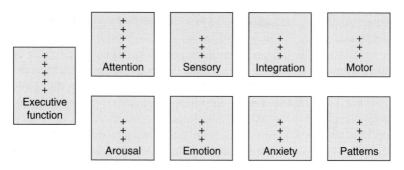

(a) Successful functioning relying on strong executive and
    attention functioning with other elements average.

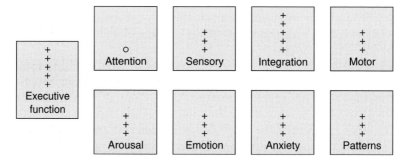

(b) Successful functioning relying on strong integration and executive
    functioning with weak attention and other elements average.

Figure 9.2 Two patterns of brain functioning representing moderate levels of success
but relying on different patterns of strength and weakness.

of strengths, the student would succeed due to learning and reasoning skills
in spite of weaknesses in attention.

Representing areas of activity in a graph such as that presented in
Figure 9.2 guides consideration of functional strengths and weaknesses in
psychotherapy clients. Such diagrams could be constructed for any
experience and could improve understanding of the experience while also
suggesting directions for intervention.

There are specific implications of the Big Picture as it is outlined
in Figure 9.1. Attention is listed first in the row of cognitive processes.
This is not because attention is always the first element activated; rather,
clinical experience has suggested that without attention the rest of the
elements often seem to collapse into a disorganized jumble no matter the

quality of processing within the elements. The very bright student with severely impaired attention has difficulty using her intelligence to solve problems. The client with impaired attention and impulse control is likely to lash out indiscriminately in the presence of powerful anger rather than activate more adaptive, thoughtful coping strategies; the emotion directly triggers motor systems without benefit of integration and executive processing.

Elements can interact in a variety of ways to yield behaviors that are quite similar. If a patient behaves impulsively, it may be because the power of the emotion is so strong, because thinking is too disorganized to support good decision-making, or because impulse control systems are so weak that the faintest inclination toward behavior is immediately and drastically expressed. If a client behaves aggressively due to psychotic confusion the appropriate interventions will be very different from interventions used to help a severely hyperactive client.

Improvements in one area may help manage or mask problems in another. If, for example, a client has a mood disorder that leads to aggressive behavior, it is possible that medical stimulation of attention systems that raises impulse control from average to high average activity levels can result in much improvement in behavioral control. This may be the case even though the underlying mood disorder has not been treated; the medicine offers the client enough "stop and think" capability so that the client can assess outcomes and control behaviors despite the presence of the mood disturbance.

Observers may falsely conclude that the success of the stimulant medication in controlling behavior "proves" that attention and impulsivity were the problems. Applying the reasoning of neuropsychological assessment to the current model, a clinician is encouraged to look beyond the impulsive outbursts to help determine whether the stimulant medication has indeed taken care of the problem. Does the client still report emotionality (high activity in affect systems) despite improved behavioral control? Does testing demonstrate psychological disorganization even though the person's scores on tasks related to concentration are quite high? The model guides the clinician toward systematically considering a number of potentially relevant aspects of cognitive and psychological functioning while assessing the client's patterns of thought, emotion, and behavior.

Elements in the bottom row can directly trigger activity in individual elements in the top row. Anger in the emotional element may directly stimulate motor systems that move a fist toward someone else's face. This may happen even though the person with the acting fist regrets the behavior later when the executive element is activated completely enough to decide what would be adaptive in the situation. LeDoux's rat demonstrating fear responses in the absence of connections between auditory receptors and auditory cortex would, if he could talk, be hard put to explain "why" the event occurred; the sensation of the bell was connected through subcortical connections directly to fear responses and motor output without the rat having the opportunity to "reflect" on the implications of the bell. It seems likely that many experiences people have and the behaviors they demonstrate are also beyond the realm of "why" in a conscious, executive processing way. Instead, motor behavior occurs when enough input into motor systems triggers neuronal action potentials connected to the fist. The input could come from executive decision-making systems acting in concert with emotion centers or, with enough intensity, the emotion centers could activate the motor system independently.

Elements of the top row can serve as specific triggers for elements in the bottom row. A student identified as having Asperger's Disorder is likely to have difficulty understanding incoming information regarding social interactions, and will therefore have difficulty predicting what will happen when he is interacting with peers. Repeated surprising negative responses from peers may lead to development of anxiety at the beginning of any social interaction. By the time the clinician meets the student, it may be difficult to identify whether the anxiety or the cognitive processing of social situations is the problem. Assessing the cues for anxiety and situations in which cognitive processing interferes with functioning can guide the clinician toward better assessment and intervention.

As presented in the current text, the Big Picture model is an extreme oversimplification. However, a strength of the model is that it encourages identification of implications that functioning in one element has for functioning in other specific elements. It also increases awareness of more complex, reciprocal interactions between such specific elements. A specific cognitive weakness within a client, for example, in verbal expression, can lead to repeated experiences of feelings of inadequacy during social interactions. Anxiety can then develop as part of the person's warning system when she is entering situations in which social judgment is likely. Social avoidance, a motor response, leads to social isolation which leads to depression, an emotional response. When the clinician encounters the depression during the intake interview, looking for sources in behavior, cognitive processing, emotion, and other elements of the system can guide the clinician toward more rapid and more integrated assessment and intervention.

Interim conclusions

The first nine chapters have presented a number of concepts related to connections between brain function and behavior, with the current chapter organizing these concepts into a framework that can guide application of these concepts to understanding how an individual functions. It is hoped the presentation has successfully walked the fine line between simplicity and complexity, thereby offering a framework for understanding brain function and the behavior of the individual that is scholarly enough without inundating and alienating the reader with the vast literature available. For readers desiring more depth or breadth of understanding, the references offered in support of concepts can provide more complete and complex insight.

The number of concepts addressed has been intentionally limited in order to avoid overwhelming clinicians who have a limited foundation in neurosciences. The depth of discussion of each concept has been limited due to the same considerations. The integration of concepts offered in the current chapter is similarly limited in complexity and intent; there are elements of brain functioning not included in the current Big Picture framework that are important to understanding how brain function affects observable, day-to-day functioning of individuals. It is hoped that despite, and because of, the limitations intentionally imposed on this presentation, the concepts and framework presented are now available to aid in understanding how people think, feel, perceive, and behave.

Throughout the previous presentation and integration of neuroscience concepts, examples have been offered hinting at the potential usefulness of applying these concepts to the process of psychotherapy. These examples have not been intended to provide a comprehensive overview of how neuroscience can be applied to psychotherapy. Rather, Part 2 of this text undertakes the presentation of a systematic application of neuroscience concepts to the psychotherapy process.

The process of psychotherapy

10

Introduction to neuroscience applications in psychotherapy

The first nine chapters presented a framework within which concepts and information related to brain function and development were considered. These ideas regarding brain development and functioning can support conceptualization and intervention in psychotherapy even though connections between specific brain processes and psychotherapy outcome have not been empirically established to a significant degree.

Neuropsychologically-based consideration of the input–process–output flow of information through the brain (Lezak, Howieson & Loring, 2004) offers basic concepts that can guide understanding of how different clients uniquely function in psychotherapy, including how clients initially perceive information, how they combine and analyze the information they receive, and how clients vary in abilities and inclinations to respond using different output systems. Recognizing the reciprocal influences of lower and higher centers in the brain (Derryberry & Tucker, 1992) can lead to better understanding of how clients experience themselves and how they can influence themselves. The concept of neural network provides an overarching context within which clients' experiences prior to and during psychotherapy can be understood and within which changes during psychological interventions can be viewed (Vaughan, 1997). Implicit and explicit memory systems can be considered to support different types of learning, experience, and change in individuals as they go through the process of psychotherapy (O'Keefe & Nadel, 1978; Schacter & Tulving, 1994). Affect systems can be viewed as especially important sources of information during psychotherapy and as influencing clients' functioning in ways that are separate from, interact with, and add to more conscious and linear logical decision-making in the brain (LeDoux, 2002; McGaugh, 2004). Anxiety is conceived as a warning system that can trigger adaptive and maladaptive responses in the presence of perceived dangerous and novel situations in a client's life (Gray & McNaughton, 2003), and in triggering such responses can strongly influence the ways maladaptive functioning in clients is supported and is amenable to improvement. Finally, brain development serves as a prism through which different elements of neural activity can be viewed as available and unfolding at different stages in a client's life (Knudsen, 2004), with implications for when to initiate what types of psychological interventions in the course of psychotherapy.

Themes inherent in development can significantly shape the manner in which clients' thoughts, emotions, and behaviors are perceived and the ways in which therapists attempt to facilitate adaptive change in children and adults. The building–pruning–myelination processes of brain development suggest differences in the implications of psychotherapy experiences for children and adults (Arnold, 1999) while also suggesting more effective ways for intervening psychotherapeutically at all stages of development. Since it appears that early experiences affect the hard wiring of the brain (Knudsen, 2004), the importance of early intervention is emphasized and the nature of intervention with adults is viewed as qualitatively different from the nature of intervention with children.

Different brain systems come on line at different stages of development (Knudsen, 2004), and as a result the relevant efficacy of psychotherapeutic techniques will vary across development. Some brain systems will fail to develop if experiences do not occur by the time developmental windows for specific systems close, and understanding of the progress of developmental windows opening and closing provides guidance during psychotherapy with regard to both when and how to intervene. Finally, activity in one brain system may profoundly alter the development of other brain systems (Andersen & Teicher, 2004; De Bellis, 2001), and recognition of interactions between systems can suggest interventions not directly relevant to the problem behaviors at hand.

Systems and patterns of brain function considered within the context of development offer an unfolding picture of the cognitive and behavioral assets available to clients of various ages with brain systems arrested in or moving through stages of development (see Figures 1.1 and 8.1). At birth, basic arousal, sensory, and motor systems are available as the underpinnings of learning through interaction with the environment. Rudimentary attention and affect systems are available, and it seems likely that basic attachment mechanisms unfold rapidly in the infant (Schore, 1994). Primitive integration systems tying in intra-modal and cross-modal information are likely present at birth but minimally developed. Kids begin to build their world using these basic tools (Teeter & Semrud-Clikeman, 1997).

Over time, the basic functions become better elaborated and new functions emerge. These developing functions affect how clients experienced and recorded earlier life events and how they can process these events at the time of psychotherapy (LeDoux, 1996). Anxiety develops, apparently as a rapid response tool for coping with threat and change (Blanchard et al., 1993). The capacity for attention improves (Casey et al., 2000; Nagy et al., 2004). Integration becomes progressively more complex in different areas of the brain, including parietal association centers and the hippocampus. Long-term memory and associated declarative memory functions emerge, supporting the development of self-awareness and contextually based organization of bits of information. Finally, more complex and effective decision-making accompanied by improved impulse control emerge to guide internal processing of information and external displays of action (Casey et al., 2000).

Biological processes within the brain have direct implications for psychotherapy. By the time a client, whether adult or child, enters psychological therapy, synapses have multiplied, strengthened, and become more efficient during development while the speed of neuronal transmission has increased (Arnold, 1999). In addition, patterns of emotion, thought, and behavior have become associated by means of repeated synaptic firing into neural networks that are conceptually the units of experience whose within-unit structure and external interactions form the bases for managing information about the world. Genetics have triggered neurological unfolding that has been influenced consistently or inconsistently by positive or negative events throughout life (Kramer, 2005).

Conceptualizations of connections between brain function and behavior can be applied directly to psychotherapy. They can provide bases for completing the intake process and initial evaluations. They can provide a framework within which psychotherapy processes can be conceived; they can guide specific interventions during therapy; and they can suggest specific tools to use during interventions. Various schools of psychotherapy can be better elaborated in light of identified relevant brain functions, and relationships between different schools of psychotherapy can be delineated in terms of an overarching framework of brain functioning. Understanding brain function can help identify the relevant strengths and weaknesses in applying each of the various psychotherapeutic approaches to interventions with a specific client.

The present outline of the connections between neuroscience and behavior provides a framework within which psychotherapy process can be conceptualized. This framework also guides development of strategies for intervention and generation of specific statements to use with clients. When various aspects of neuroscience processing were less well understood, ideas regarding brain activity could occasionally be used to fill in gaps of understanding not covered by more traditional theories of intervention used within an eclectic framework. Increasingly neuroscience conceptualization has the potential to usefully "invade" all aspects of therapy, now reaching the point that from the initial assessment through the conclusion of therapy, recognition and application of knowledge of brain function can be an integral aspect of intervening.

In some therapy cases the brain may remain a background guide to decision-making for the therapist but never be part of overt discussion with the patient. In such situations the therapist is guided to select one or another of the traditional psychotherapy intervention strategies based on understanding of the client developed within the larger context of brain function. However, it may be the therapist never refers to the brain because the explanations offered by traditional theory provide adequate explanation, direction, and motivation in treatment. For example, following cognitive behavioral therapy guidelines, global, negative self-statements regarding the client's own qualities may be targeted and then addressed using strategies for replacing these self-statements with statements that focus on positive strengths and positive possibilities (Beck, 1976). No reference to the brain need be made, and positive improvement in client functioning may be obtained. In the early stages of developing the current framework of brain–psychotherapy interaction, the author found such cases to be common; however, as knowledge regarding brain function has become better elaborated and has seemed to contribute more details to the understanding of the process of psychotherapy, moving through therapy without referring to the brain has become progressively less typical.

In the second part of this book, applications to psychotherapy process will be considered in light of how various elements of neuroscience functioning contribute to the therapy process. Specific implications for the intake process will be outlined. The neural network concept provides the primary context within which brain science ideas are applied, so it will be presented next. The contributions of affect systems are an integral aspect of the neural network and will be presented as part of the neural network model. The implications of theories of memory will then be considered, with particular emphasis on the nature of change over the course of psychotherapy. The implications of the Gray model of anxiety will be outlined. Direct effects of the overall brain science model on interactions with clients will then be considered. Finally, relationships between the brain science framework and other theories of psychotherapy and psychiatric intervention will be discussed.

11

Intake and assessment

Neuroscience concepts can influence what information is gathered during the intake process. Various schools of psychotherapy support obtaining information in various specific areas of psychological and personal functioning, but consideration of brain function encourages collection of a broader range of information while maintaining awareness of how the various pieces of information relate to each other. Psychodynamic (Fenichel, 1945) and object relations (Mahler *et al.*, 1975) theories emphasize gathering information regarding the family dynamics within which the patient developed. Behavior analysis (Bellack *et al.*, 1990) emphasizes the identification of environmental stimulus events, description of problem behaviors, and delineation of consequences of behavior. Traditional cognitive behavioral therapy encourages the identification of irrational thoughts that occur in response to specific events and ideas (Beck, 1976). A brain-based model of psychotherapy directs the therapist to gather information related to each of these areas so a full understanding of brain-based behaviors related to problematic functioning can be obtained. A brain-based model provides for identification of all possible contributors to the current shape and function of the brain, and calls for as complete an understanding as possible of how these contributors interact.

The intake interview designed to support a neuroscience-based model of intervention includes information from the following areas:

- Genetics
- Biological events
- Early interpersonal patterns
- Later interpersonal patterns
- History of family structure and events
- Current behavioral functioning

Information from these areas might be collected in support of therapy based on any of the various schools of intervention, but using the brain to guide assessment leads to changes in the process of gathering intake information as well as in the content of intake interviews.

The present discussion will focus on identifying how the nature of the intake process shifts when the brain is the underlying source of structure. Aspects of the intake process that seem not to differ significantly from what would be obtained without the introduction of brain concepts will not be addressed. In order to make clear the reasons for gathering specific information during the intake process, discussion of the intake interview will often expand into discussion of how questions addressed during the intake process are related to assessment and to specific aspects of psychotherapy intervention. It should be noted that the intake outline presented here is arranged based on the chronology of influence on the patient rather than on the flow of the interview itself.

Broadly conceived, using a brain-based approach introduces an intervening variable that mediates the ways elements identified during assessment influence the patient's problem behaviors (see Figure 11.1). In the course of a traditional approach to assessment, identification of symptoms guides the evaluator to a diagnosis that suggests specific treatment and may lead to identification of other symptoms. When specific brain functions and brain systems are identified during the assessment process, connections between various possible diagnoses can be more

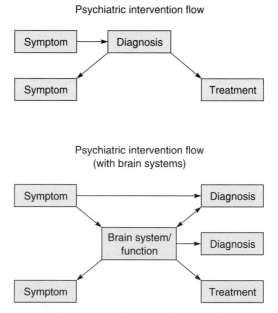

Figure 11.1 Diagnosis and treatment with and without considering brain function.

effectively considered, nuances of functioning within specific diagnoses can be better identified, and connections between assessment and treatment can be more directly established. Furthermore, such an approach to assessment facilitates establishing interactions between genetic background, physical influences, and interpersonal experiences during the development of particular patterns of adaptive behavior and pathology.

Genetics

When brain functioning is central in assessment and treatment, identification of possible genetic contributions to neural development and activity becomes critical. Focus on genetics, including family mental health history, also provides examples of how the introduction of the brain as an intervening variable affects assessment.

Assessment of depression provides an example of the impact of considering genetic contributions as well as of the effect of considering brain systems as an element of the evaluation. Without considering the brain, identification of a family history of depression would be considered to directly influence prediction of what behaviors are likely to be present in a person's current functioning. A family history of depression increases the likelihood that the patient will experience depression. This connection has the potential to remain an abstract conception, but when the intervening variable of brain systems, including neurotransmitters and brain systems involved, is included, awareness of implications is heightened. Genetically based vulnerability to "kindling" of depression through repeated episodes of depression can be more clearly understood when the concepts of neural networks and sensitization of neural connections (Kandel *et al.*, 2000b, pp. 1248–52) are used to explain that bouts of depression can become more frequent and severe over time. Reference to brain activity and lack of activity may help explain the effects of depression on concentration (Mayberg *et al.*, 2002), and thereby help explain effects on school and work performance. Or, effects of a parent's depression on the developing brains of children exposed to the depressed parent can be better understood when the interplay between the child's genetic inclination to depression and the depressed parent's lack of reciprocal interaction behavior is explained (Dawson *et al.*, 1999; Rutter, 2005). In each of these cases, understanding is likely to be improved when consideration of the mediating element of brain systems involved is incorporated into the assessment and conceptualization of genetic influences on the depressive process.

Recognition of genetic contributions to a child's current functioning can lead to better understanding of a child's neurological processing. For example, if a learning disability is present in the child being assessed, the question, "Is there anyone in the family who thinks in the way this child does?" can lead to identification of a possible genetic basis for a brain wiring pattern mediating the disability. The question also suggests that the similar adult may have particularly valuable observations to make regarding how a brain with this structure takes in information and solves problems. The similar adult can be asked to reflect on and describe the adult's own strategies for coping with the learning disability shared by the parent and the child. In this manner, a brain with the same deficits but with active frontal lobes (that is, capacity to monitor and analyze) can assist in identifying ways the child can most effectively use a brain wired in the same fashion. This consideration of brain elements involved is much different from simply checking off on a list the probability that this is a genetic rather than an environmentally based learning problem.

Biological events

Consideration of the brain emphasizes exploration of biological events beyond what would be emphasized by traditional theories. Prenatal events, the birth process, and subsequent physical trauma affecting the brain can all change how the client's brain processes information, arousal, and emotion.

Assessment of prenatal events, especially chemical exposure during gestation, is completed with particular thought to the effects on migration of neurons during gestation. Problems during childhood years with cognitive integration and arousal modulation secondary to cocaine or alcohol abuse during pregnancy are highlighted (Guerri, 1998; Jacobson, 1998). There are indications maternal stress contributes to alterations in temperament of offspring due to the influence of the stress response on brain development during gestation (Hayashi et al., 1998; Kofman, 2002; Watson et al., 1999). The potential for delayed expression of problems based on disruption of migration is also emphasized by focus on potential biological insults to brain development. Researchers studying schizophrenia have theorized that disruption of migration of neurons into hippocampal integration areas may occur during gestation but not be significantly expressed in disruption of thought and behavior until late adolescence because the relevant neurons do not typically become integrated into overall brain function until that point in development (Kotrla et al., 1997).

Hypoxia during delivery has effects that can be expressed in immediate changes in brain functioning as well as in a delayed fashion. Hypoxia results in the death of cells (Shalak & Perlman, 2004). The hippocampus is particularly vulnerable to the effects of hypoxia but, at more severe levels, lack of oxygen can damage cells throughout the brain and interfere with related functioning (Saper, 2000). When damage is mild and apparently restricted to the hippocampus, the effects may not be seen until a child is 8 or 9 years old. This is because the brain processes on which cognitive processing rests during the early years tend to be implicit in nature, relying more on the influence of experience on simple connections between neurons throughout the brain rather than on activity in the hippocampus and other integration areas. Education from kindergarten through second grade (serving ages 5 through 7 years) tends to focus on the learning of facts, while after that point learning becomes progressively more integrative in nature. Since the hippocampus is a center for establishing complex interrelationships between facts, the deficiencies in capacity for integration do not become evident until the child reaches the age and level of education at which such integration would be required; that is, when the hippocampus would be needed for appropriate functioning.

When hippocampal damage due to hypoxia is expressed in limited capacity to integrate information, there are shifts in patterns of coping throughout life. In therapy, a client who has experienced such an event will be more likely to learn through repeated experience rather than through development of insight, and it appears such a client functions better when given templates or lists of steps for dealing with situations rather than through being taught how to generate new responses to novel problems. Behavioral or cognitive behavioral techniques would seem likely to be more effective for such clients than would psychodynamic, insight-oriented therapy. In the workplace, such a client will do better in a job that relies on stable routines rather than on creative problem-solving in the face of new difficulties. In school, students with impairment related to hypoxia at birth will work better when given templates, that is, specific step-by-step guidelines, for completing writing and mathematical tasks. The relevance of identifying such early experiences becomes clear when the implications for subsequent functioning mediated by damage to this area of the brain are understood.

Physical damage to the brain after birth can have a variety of effects on the developing brain depending on the location of the damage, the extent of the damage, and the age at which the damage occurred. There are indications that when focal (localized and limited) brain damage occurs in the first year of life due to disruption in blood flow to a specific area of the cortex the brain can recover to near the level of normal functioning, likely due to the young brain's plasticity, that is, ready availability to change (Levin, 2003). It appears recovery occurs because the brain is flexible enough to include new parts of the brain in carrying out the same behavioral task.

When the brain is battered due to being shaken, dropped, or banged into the dash board of a car, resulting damage can be both obvious and not so obvious. Effects can include brain damage that can observably disrupt specific behavioral functions depending on the specific location of the blow to the brain. However, such trauma to the brain may also damage long axons connecting various areas of the brain; some of the effects of such damage may not be observable until the child's brain reaches later stages of development that depend heavily on integrating information from throughout the brain.

Current evidence suggests that when a brain injury is mild, localized, and occurs when the child is younger, recovery may be more complete than when the child is older. However, there are also indications that if brain damage is severe and is accompanied by damage to long axons that typically become involved in the integration of information across areas of the brain, recovery may be poor even if the child is an infant at the time of the damage. It appears the infant brain's plasticity may help the brain recover from mild but not severe damage encountered at a young age (Levin, 2003). Maintaining a brain-based focus on therapy reminds the therapist of the importance of such damage to current functioning and future development, and also guides the evaluator to be more specific with regard to what parts of the brain were injured at what point in development so the best understanding possible regarding implications for cognitive and behavioral functioning can be developed.

Seizures can affect cognitive functioning directly by disrupting functioning at the moment of the seizure, by disrupting cognitive functioning over a period of time while the brain recovers from the seizure, and by causing permanent damage over the long term to specific or broad areas of the brain (Westbrook, 2000). Identifying the age of occurrence, localization, and severity of seizures can contribute to understanding what aspects of development have likely been disrupted with what implications for functioning. It appears the earlier seizures occur, the more severe the impairment in cognitive functioning is likely to be. Medications prescribed to control seizures can themselves result in disruptions in cognitive processing including reduced sustained attention, memory, and verbal fluency, as well as disruption in mood (Howieson et al., 2004). It seems likely that reductions in functioning due to medication reflect reduction in brain activity that may contribute to less effective synaptogenesis, arborization, and pruning.

Impaired physical capabilities such as the ability to see can contribute to disruption in development of other brain capacities (Freedman, 1981). Studies of blind children indicated that the parents of these children tend to quickly reduce their involvement with their children because of the lack of response to visual interaction. Whereas it initially appeared that the visual deficit itself contributed to development of inappropriate behaviors, it became clear after study that the lack of reciprocal interaction was the actual source of behavioral deterioration. When parents were taught to interact reciprocally in the absence of response to visual activity, the children's behaviors were found to be much more appropriate and well-modulated. It seems likely that underlying brain mechanisms associated with stress modulation and attachment had been developing inappropriately in the absence of an ongoing experience of reciprocal emotional–social interactions with a caretaker (Schore, 1994).

Physical disorders that include persistent distress that is unresponsive to the ministrations of caretakers seem likely to have the potential to disrupt brain development and personal functioning as well (Desantis *et al.*, 2004), and therefore need to be identified during assessment. Brain development depends on the consistent simultaneous firing of neurons in order to strengthen synapses and maintain neuronal connections through the period of pruning. If a baby experiences chronic pain that cannot be soothed by a caretaker, then the baby does not experience repeated rehearsal of pain leading to crying leading to the appearance of the parent leading to soothing. It therefore seems likely that basic neural networks related to both attachment and sense of efficacy would be weak or absent and therefore not available as the child continues to grow.

Some children are hypersensitive to all types of stimulation including sound and touch. It is surmised that if most sounds are startling, whether the concurrent situation is actually threatening or not, then the child is likely to develop hypersensitive startle responses similar to those experienced in abused children because of the unpredictability, frequency, and intensity of the sounds. For children who are overly sensitive to touch and therefore avoid it, opportunities to establish attachment through the soothing of touch are lost, with implications for the subsequent loss of opportunity to obtain social reinforcement and support.

Interpersonal influences

Most theories of psychotherapy intervention include some type of focus on previous history of interpersonal interactions; social learning theory (Bandura, 1977) and objections relations theory (Mahler *et al.*, 1975) are examples. However, consideration of the brain as a mediating variable shifts the focus of such consideration to some degree. Consideration of the brain guides focus during intake to a wider variety of types of social influence, to variations based on stage of development, and to the effects of social experiences on the brain's ability to carry out tasks not typically considered to be social in nature.

A neuropsychological perspective and the concept of neural networks combine to offer a broad framework within which interpersonal interactions can be assessed and categorized. Traditional behavioral theories would guide intake assessment toward identifying current behavioral responses to current social stimuli. Such an assessment would downplay the importance of cognitions, self-statements, or history of attachment. Assessment based on cognitive behavioral theory would evaluate behavioral patterns addressed during a typical assessment based on behavior therapy, and would also emphasize conscious self-statements regarding relationships. A psychodynamic assessment would emphasize relationship history but might disregard assessment of current social skills.

A brain-based assessment would examine a wider range of factors related to interpersonal functioning. Current behavioral and cognitive behavioral themes related to interpersonal functioning would be assessed as part of a brain-based assessment. The quality of interpersonal bonds established throughout life would be emphasized (Knudsen, 2004). The history of relationships over the span of development would help identify potential sources of distress as well as security in the interpersonal realm. The effects of early social experience on attachment processes, which would likely be stored in implicit memory systems, would be addressed (Schore, 1994). In looking at these early processes the client's currently available interpersonal resources could be identified. Cognitive pathways for receiving and expressing social connection would be evaluated; for example, the relative strengths of verbal and non-verbal processing would be determined. The brain-based assessment of interpersonal functioning includes specific elements addressed by many traditional theories while adding understanding derived from recognition of the influences of stages of brain development on integrating interpersonal experiences.

Assessment of the child's experiences during the first 5 years of life is important to include in an intake focused on understanding the client's brain development. Brain development during the first 5 years of life is characterized by rapid proliferation of axons, dendrites, and synapses (Casey et al., 2000). The extent of this proliferation is strongly influenced by the amount of stimulation available in the environment (Bennett et al., 1964; Greenough et al., 1987), and development of patterns of brain activity is likely to be shaped by the nature of the young child's experiences (Ford, 2005).

Animal studies have shown that experimental rats raised in highly stimulating environments have heavier cortices than rats raised in non-stimulating environments. Amounts of dendritic and synaptic material present in the brains of these rats are correspondingly higher.

The visual system of the cat offers further evidence that stimulation from the external environment clearly alters the physical structure of the brain. Post mortem examination has revealed that if one eye of a cat has been sutured closed during early development, neurons in the visual cortex display a pattern of alternating robust development and atrophy that can be visually observed (Hubel & Wiesel, 1970).

Because early brain development is strongly influenced by the environment, it is important to assess the consistency of social interactions experienced by the child and to assess the qualitative characteristics of these interactions. Children raised by substance abusing parents who periodically abandoned them, who failed to respond to the their needs in predictable ways, or who inflicted unpredictable and severe pain would be expected to have fewer and weaker neural connections since strength of connections is based on connected neurons repeatedly firing at the same time (Teicher et al., 2004). Or, in the case of regularly inflicted pain, it is likely that connections would be established that reflect the expectation that painful events rather than soothing events will occur.

It has been suggested that the soothing offered by nurturing parents helps develop children's internal capacity to soothe themselves and manage arousal. This aspect of brain development would be expected to be impaired in children lacking such experiences (Glaser, 2000). Agitation, low frustration tolerance, and limited capacity for reasoning would likely characterize such children, and would reflect the wiring of the brain.

The experiences of children who have not been neglected or abused, that is, who have been raised normally, are also assumed to shape the synaptogenesis, arborization, and pruning of neurons and the concomitant development of neural networks, albeit in more developmentally normal and adaptive ways. Therefore, understanding as completely as possible the early family experiences of each child being assessed will offer insights regarding brain development and capacity for relationships whether or not traumatic events have occurred during development.

It appears that the effects of early family relationships on the brain are not accompanied by conscious memories before the age of 3 or 4 years. There are indications that this is due to lack of maturation of neural centers that support explicit, declarative integration of incoming information (Bauer, 2004) and subsequent long term memory storage (Squire et al., 1993). Rather, procedural or implicit memory processes will encode these experiences in the connections between various sensory, motor, affect, and integration neurons, establishing neural networks that then trigger associations and emotions even if the associations cannot be explained. The nature of the neural systems available at the time of encoding will influence the child's processing of interpersonal relationships at any given point in development, and will affect the way in which such information is subsequently recalled regardless of the extent of eventual development in explicit memory systems. At the same time, the development of brain structures underlying memory systems will continue to be modified by the very experiences they encode over the course of development (Ford, 2005).

Pertinent information to be obtained regarding early family experiences includes the emotional states of the parents. For example, the emotional state of the mother during a client's early years should be investigated because a depressed mother's neglect can have significant negative effects on a child's development (Glaser, 2000). Extended separations during the first several years of life can have deleterious effects on development, as demonstrated in studies by Bowlby (1973). This is true even if the reason for the separation, such as an extended vacation, is a positive one in the eyes of the parents.

The level of availability of other parenting figures should be noted. It may be that even though one parent was unavailable to the child, there were other parenting figures who offered the child enough stability to develop adequate attachment. Furthermore, Schore (1994) has suggested that the availability of a second parenting figure may offer opportunities for development of a second set of elements of attachment at a later stage in brain development, thereby offering a sense of security combined with a greater sense of safety. The availability or lack of availability of such secondary attachment figures may have subtle effects. For example, a student reported that he had been able to develop a positive bond with his father even though his father worked in a foreign country separate from the child for the first 7 years of life; however, later in the conversation it was reported that the student had changed his last name out of convenience when he reached the age of majority, a change that suggested attachment bonds were weak despite the lack of overt distress.

The character of the child's own initial behavior patterns and temperament should be ascertained since some children contribute to poor bonding because their own behaviors interfere with the parents' attempts to bond (Freedman, 1981). When the parent says the child was "...evil from the day she was born!" it can be surmised that the experiences encoded into neural connections and networks for this child did not reflect positive interactions with parenting figures. This assumption would likely be true whether the evaluation of the child as "evil" was a distortion by the parent or an assessment consistent with deficits in the child's functioning.

It is useful to know about other events in the parents' lives during the early years of development, since events such as the death of a parent's parent may disrupt the availability of the parent to the child. The birth of siblings, particularly those immediately before and immediately after the person being assessed, may also influence the experiences and thus brain development of the client.

Information regarding interpersonal relationship patterns should be gathered regarding development beyond the first several years of life. This information should be tempered by the understanding that as development progresses the tendencies will be for the brain's hard wiring to be less strongly influenced by experiences at the same time that the client will have greater awareness of influential events that have occurred. If the father becomes more available to and positive with a child after a career change occurs when the child is 13 years old, it is assumed that the previously developed declarative and non-declarative neural networks that include images of an emotionally unavailable father who was pressured and unpredictable are likely to continue contributing significantly to the child's interpretations of experiences. However, if the father made the same change when the child was 4 years old, the likelihood is that declarative and procedural memories including positive affective connections with images of the father would be stronger and leave the child more likely to interpret as sincere the father's positive interventions when the child is 13 year old.

All external events and the reactions to them described by the client need to be interpreted in light of the developmental stage of the person at the time of the experience. This is because the level of brain development and the concomitant nature of cognitive processing will strongly affect what the client perceives and how it is recorded in the brain. A client may, because of the concrete, self-referential nature of psychological processing at that age, remember violence between parents when the child was 4 or 5 years old as being caused by the client, when in fact events were triggered by factors of which the child had no knowledge. The 4-year-old observing violence is likely to record information as direct procedural connections between affect and sensory systems, and to have little ability to apply conscious, self-soothing strategies that would need to be coordinated with frontal lobe executive systems.

On the other hand, a 15-year-old will likely remember the same violence with greater capacity to integrate contextual cues, such as the fact the father had been caught having an affair with another woman and had subsequently threatened the mother with financial abandonment. The 15-year-old will also be more likely than the 4-year-old to record information in the relatively well-developed frontal-hippocampal declarative memory system in addition to procedural memory systems. In addition, when family violence is experienced by the client at age 15 years, the frontal lobes will be available to modulate the affect experienced at the time the information is being "recorded" so the experience is less likely to be recorded as emotionally overwhelming.

When information regarding family functioning before the age of 3 years is not available, the memories of the client dating from after the first several years of life may be suspected, with some risk of being wrong, to be congruent with the nature of family functioning before that time. The assumption is that patterns tend to remain the same over time. It is always possible that the changes in the family situation led to changes in the way the parents interacted with the child over time, so perceptions of the family derived from experiences later in the developmental process may in fact not be the same as those experienced earlier. A sudden increase in financial stresses on the family requiring the mother to begin working when the child is 5 years old could lead to increased unavailability or rejecting reactiveness on the part of the parents during parenting interventions after such a change. Memory of these rejecting experiences by the child in later years may not adequately represent the level of positive attachment the client is able to make if the years prior to the change were characterized by the establishment of soothing, consistent emotional bonds with the mother.

Furthermore, the nature of the client's contributions to the situation will change over the course of development, and it will be important to keep that in mind when projecting later patterns into the earlier years of development. If a client describes experiences as a 6-year-old that reflect the child's conscious choice to avoid the parent because of a parent's anger in response to the child's impulsive behaviors, the temptation is to assume that such a pattern of coping was also present before age 6 years. However, if the same experiences occurred before integration capacity and long-term memory processes were well-developed, primary elements in the pattern are likely to involve procedural, non-declarative neural connections characterized by an absence of planful response. The impulsive 2-year-old may not develop a conscious plan for avoidance, and will instead have automatic responses such as crying or running away. The pattern being laid down at the time would thus have a different form and therefore different impact on subsequent development than running away at age 6 years.

Summarizing the assessment of a client's history of interpersonal relationships, the intake process is guided by consideration of brain development to focus on the influences of early interpersonal interaction patterns on attachment, affect modulation, and neural network patterns. Identifying the earliest interpersonal experiences is assumed to be important in understanding the procedural memory connections that have been established between sensory systems, arousal systems, action systems, and affect. Goals of intake and assessment are to identify contributors to implicit memory neural networks of which the client may have no awareness as well as contributors to declarative memory systems of which the client will have varying levels of awareness.

Current functioning

The details related to current functioning collected during an intake founded on brain development are not much different from information collected during intake processes based on traditional theoretical models of psychotherapy (see Figure 11.1). However, the reliance on brain function as an intervening variable continues to be present as a contextual element subtly influencing clinical understanding. Behaviors are assumed to reflect underlying neural capacities, and during the intake process the implications of neural capacities identified as possibly supporting a specific behavior may go beyond ties typically made between one type of behavior and another.

The Big Picture model (see Figure 9.1) supports such alterations in assessment of various symptom patterns. Problems with affective dyscontrol would be considered in light of the possibilities of problems with arousal centers, emotion centers, or impulse control centers. If problems were with arousal centers, they would be displayed in the course of a variety of positive and negative events, some of which could include excitement or agitation rather than negative emotions. If problems were with emotion centers, the symptoms would tend to be in situations associated with specific negative emotions such as loss, rejection, or fear. If problems were with impulse control systems, problems would be displayed in the absence of cues for emotion, frustration, or excitement, and would appear to be associated with overly impulsive expressions of average mood or arousal. Considering a different symptom pattern, problems with distractibility in the school setting would prompt assessment of behaviors reflecting the overall input–process–output system, and might therefore lead to the identification of problems with verbal auditory processing rather than distractibility as the source of the problem.

In addition to simply offering extra hypotheses regarding the reasons for the presentation of specific symptoms, consideration of brain functioning can also support better understanding of interactions between various problem areas. For example, sudden presentation of problems with mood and affective dyscontrol during third and fourth grade, (ages 8 through 9 years) could be the result of increasing frustration associated with problems with cognitive integration related to hypoxia at birth interacting with a genetically-based mood disorder identified through family history. The decision regarding whether attention deficit is a problem warranting immediate intervention in a younger child may change when it is considered whether attention problems will significantly limit the neuronal repetitions necessary for optimal development of integration areas.

Current intake procedures based on traditional theories of psychotherapy continue to offer valid structure and guidance to the assessment process.

However, consideration of underlying neural substrates of behavior appears likely to support generation of additional hypotheses related to the origins of specific behavior. Focus on brain systems also appears to offer a framework for initial assessment during intake that is both broader and more complete than that offered by any single traditional theory currently extant. Intake and assessment based on brain functioning provide the groundwork for applying to psychotherapy neuroscience concepts related to neural networks, affect, memory, learning, and anxiety.

12

Neural networks in therapy

Each experience, whether current event or memory, is assumed to consist of a unique network of neurons from many parts of the brain: a neural network. Sensory systems, motor tracts, brain stem arousal systems, affect centers, hippocampal integration centers, anxiety responses, and frontal executive centers are all likely represented in a given neural network. These pieces of the neural network provide the framework through which experiences observable to the client, the therapist, and other people interacting with the client can be understood. Such experiences include the phenomena of cognition and affect, expressed behavior, shifts in attention, experience and demonstration of anxiety, and physiological responding. A specific network is likely to become active when enough of the neurons of which it is composed are stimulated at the same time. In a complementary fashion, other networks that share neurons with the network of immediate interest are likely to be triggered when enough shared neurons are simultaneously firing.

Using neural network concepts as needed

Psychotherapy cases can often be adequately represented by traditional psychotherapy theories. In such cases, interventions can be conceived and described in terms of the traditional theory being used, and neuroscience conceptualizations would be included only when they offer additional insight to the traditional theory being used. Consequently, time would not be spent helping the client develop an overall or in-depth understanding of the neural network model.

For example, in the case of a simple fear of heights in which family history is positive for genetically based anxiety and in which exploration during intake has revealed no psychodynamic patterns supporting the fear, typical progressive exposure with relaxation would be used (Wolpe, 1958).

Only minimal references to brain processes would be offered. Development of relaxation skills would be initiated with an explanation that therapy will work toward pairing sensory cues related to height with the emotional and physiological state of being relaxed. It would be pointed out that relaxation impedes the development of a high anxiety state accompanied by brain stem activity that floods the brain with neurotransmitters that interfere with brain function and are experienced as a high state of arousal. A progressive exposure plan would be developed whereby the client is able to maintain a relatively relaxed state while experiencing progressively more intense cues associated with height. Connections between the cues and anxiety are expected to become habituated because of the nature of anxiety related neural transmission whereby the transmitters needed to support the experience of anxiety are used up during exposure, and the anxiety is no longer present. Simultaneously, the cues are paired with the relaxed state. Following multiple repetitions, a neural network that pairs height cues with relaxation replaces a neural network that previously paired height cues with panic.

In one specific case of the treatment of fear of heights, when treatment progressed toward more intense height-related experiences, such as looking over the edge of a six story parking garage, it became clear that sensations of vertigo were part of the trigger for the neural network of anxiety associated with height. It was therefore explained that a natural internal reaction, vertigo, experienced by a large number of people was part of the trigger for the anxiety reaction. A goal was identified whereby the client practiced experiencing vertigo without going on to experience panic. Habituation to vertigo subsequently developed.

In treating test anxiety, initial assessment during intake may indicate either that complex psychodynamic patterns are not involved, or that because of the limited capacities of the client it is likely to be more effective to focus on an aspect of overall functioning that has limited scope. A problem-focused intervention addressing test anxiety would then be developed. Initial phases of treatment for test anxiety would be similar to the classic behavioral treatment for fear of heights just described: relaxation skills training would be offered. However, more complete discussion of the nature of neural networks would be relevant in order to give the client better focus on the task of disrupting the onset of test anxiety. A general description of a neural network would be offered followed by a description of how one network can interfere with the functioning of another because of the brain's tendency to focus on one topic, i.e. network, at a time. Also described would be how two different networks, one related to test topic content and one related to fear of failure, could trigger each other because of the shared "node" of taking a test on the content material. Test taking is conceived as being part of the test material network as well as part of the fear of failure network. If one network is active and in awareness, other networks tend to be less active and therefore out of the realm of attention. The client would be given instructions in shifting attention from the fear network to the content material network.

One intervention suggested by such a view of brain functioning is a thought substitution procedure (Borkovec *et al.*, 1983; Mahoney, 1974) designed to activate a positive network rather than shut down a negative network. The example of "Don't think about red cars" might be offered in order to make it clear that every statement against red cars includes red cars, while every description of a substitute image of hiking in the Rocky Mountains leads to the disappearance of the red car image. The client would be given instructions regarding how to activate the content networks related to the test material. If the example test is regarding the history of Texas, the client would be encouraged to see a picture of the Alamo in her head, to recall the teacher talking about the Alamo, to imagine writing notes about the Alamo, to recall a visit to the Alamo and remember what the stones felt like, and to remember the words of the text in the section of the book about the Alamo. Rather than trying to remember the specific date of the battle asked for in the test, the goal of focus is to activate the whole network or set of networks related to the Alamo, with the idea that the date is more likely to pop into awareness if enough of the rest of the "Alamo network" is activated.

The idea that the network consists of elements from various parts of the brain guides the therapist to include as many brain systems as possible during the activation of a network, including sensory, motor, and integration systems. This is an example of priming in which focus on a type of material increases the likelihood that the networks related to the consciously primed one will operate faster and with greater vigor (Posner & Raichle, 1994). The client would be told that slipping back to the fear of failure network is likely since the setting of test taking has multiple cues that are part of that network; for example, encountering a question, the answer to which is not immediately known. Remembering the intrusive red car, the client is encouraged to breathe calmly in order to relax, and then to work yet again on the various strategies for activating the substitute neural network related to test content. It would be pointed out during the therapy session that focusing on failure will not increase the likelihood of doing better on the test; only focusing on content material increases the likelihood of doing better on the test. It would also be pointed out that focusing on "success" or a high grade does not activate neural networks related to the Alamo; in fact, focusing on success is likely to activate judgment networks that are likely to revive the anxiety regarding failure that impairs functioning. Rather than focus on failure or success, the client would be encouraged to perceive the grade as a secondary result following the most complete activation of the content networks possible. The only value of focusing on the grade is to generate motivation, and increasing motivation is most valuable when deciding to study, not during study or during the test. Focusing on content elements that can activate the neural networks related to content is presented as the primary goal of interventions to manage test anxiety.

Viewed from the perspective of influencing the brain, problem-focused interventions such as those just described have ramifications beyond habituation of specific maladaptive networks and priming and rehearsal of adaptive ones. First, taking the step to initiate a shift in focus is assumed to simultaneously activate executive centers in the frontal lobes while also activating networks related to self-image. Intervening successfully at a lower level, that is, at the level of choosing to activate more positive networks, is likely to result in the pairing of feelings of success with positive decision making and positive images of the self as effective. In addition, some writers (Derryberry & Tucker, 1992) have referred to the presence of separate brain systems mediating active intervention and passive avoidance. The more times the active coping systems are stimulated as part of networks related to problem resolution, the more likely it is that proactive coping will be activated in the future when the client encounters problems. Indirectly, the self has been altered.

Elaborating on neural network concepts

Psychotherapy cases can be so complex and obscure that the underlying bases for maladaptive functioning remain unclear, and it is therefore difficult to initiate effective change. Often the client's reports of internal experiences are not congruent with observed external behaviors. The client's reports and the understanding gained by the therapist do not yield an understanding of the processes at work. A client might report that when he begins to feel close to a heterosexual partner he always begins to behave in ways that disrupt the relationship. Or the client might report having panic attacks for no apparent reason and subsequently missing work on a regular basis. At such times it becomes useful to discuss neural networks with the client in greater detail in order to facilitate problem identification and movement toward change.

The first step in such a discussion is to propose that each reaction the client has is connected within the brain to other elements of functioning. The nature of neural networks is then described in a way similar to the description offered above when working with a person experiencing test anxiety. More of the ramifications of the neural network model are then discussed. Parts of the network may remain out of awareness, and it will be helpful to make more parts of the network clear. The network, including its unrecognized parts, is likely connected to other networks, and these networks may be primed into awareness by the onset of the poorly defined network that includes the current problem. The client is then encouraged to "notice what pops into your head" since the thoughts that pop into a person's head while discussing problematic issues are likely to be related to problematic issues by way of neural network connections yet to be defined. The client and the therapist may then reflect further on ideas and images that continue to "pop" into awareness, and eventually a persistent theme may be identified. The theme may be an emotion or a pattern of behavior or a memory from earlier in development.

In the case of a client sabotaging heterosexual relationships for no good reason, a stream of images might flow from "a Golden Retriever" to "petting and hugging the dog" to "the dog baring its teeth" to "a Doberman Pinscher snarling with teeth bared. . ." Further exploration might lead to images of the client being loved supportively by his mother and later being slapped and abandoned by his mother. In this example, beginning with focus on a roadblock in therapy, following the connections of the neural network have led to identification of networks related to a history that helps to account for the distress and maladaptive behaviors that were previously not understood.

Details of the process of exploring the neural network can be addressed with the client as needed and appropriate. The client is encouraged *not* to ask "Why does this response occur?" Why questions are viewed as activating frontal brain systems designed to guide access to the rest of the consciously accessible brain, and such systems are likely to block the discovery of memories that have not yet been connected to declarative memory systems and executive functioning (see Squire *et al.*, 1993). The goal of following connections in the neural network is to allow memories to unfold that are primarily procedural rather than declarative in nature. The client is encouraged to allow silly thoughts or thoughts that suggest weakness or ineffectuality to emerge. Since the brain does not connect pieces of information in ways that make overt sense to us as observers, some thoughts or images may seem silly. Such thoughts are described as giving clues about how connections are arranged rather than as defining who the client is as a person. Irrational thought patterns, that is, maladaptive parts of a neural network, may be uncovered during exploration of the neural network, and this uncovering is likely to open the door for improvement. Understanding connections within the neural network is likely to lead to development of more effective ways of dealing with life and is therefore likely to end up giving the person an increased sense of power rather than a more limited one.

The Big Picture model (Figure 9.1) offers a visual representation of the relationship between various elements of brain function and unique neural network patterns established due to particular patterns of experience in a client's past. The model can guide the therapist's conceptualization of the role of such patterns in activating a client's functioning, and can also be shared directly with the client in order to facilitate the process of developing awareness of connections as they unfold. Various other specific elements of the Big Picture model may regularly influence the client's functioning when there is no apparent pattern of experience to account for such influence. For example, due to a family history of anxiety, a client may overreact to external situations whether there is an pattern of past experience to support such reaction or not. In such cases, a pattern of experience in the past is not considered to be the primary influence. However, when patterns of past experience contribute to current triggering of other elements of the Big Picture in a repeated fashion, such patterns become the focus of consideration during treatment.

"Following connections within the neural network" is extremely similar to free association in psychodynamic therapy processes. It is also very much in line with Shapiro's process of following connections in Eye Movement Desensitization and Reprocessing (EMDR) (Shapiro, 1995). In fact, it appears that the brain processes underlying each of these interventions are likely to be the same. When compared to free association in the context of psychodynamic psychotherapy, outlining the neural network offers a more concrete explanation than that of "allowing the unconscious to emerge". Offering guidance for exploring neural networks is conceived as allowing the client to maintain a greater sense of personal control and effectiveness than the psychodynamic admonition to allow the unconscious to emerge. Letting go of personal control is not viewed as being requisite for exploration of connections.

Compared to the process outlined by Shapiro, following the neural network implies collaboration with the therapist rather than giving up control to the therapist who assumes a lead role in taking the client through the exploration of connections between one experience and another during EMDR. Following the neural network is also viewed as being useful in gaining understanding of any experience, not just the deprogramming of previous trauma. Exploring neural networks can therefore be useful as a tool for the client to use independently in life, and can be a tool at multiple points in therapy.

A specific implication of the neural network concept can guide the therapist regarding how to intervene in therapy during exploration of issues. The network representing a given experience is assumed to consist of neurons from many parts of the brain. An experience being addressed in therapy likely includes, for example, neurons from sensory systems, motor systems, affect systems, visual-spatial integration areas, verbal integration areas, and frontal decision making areas. The network can therefore be accessed by initiating firing of neurons in any of these areas. The therapist can ask the client to notice feelings that are currently being experienced, and then notice what other ideas pop into the client's head while experiencing the feeling. The client can be asked to "relive" a related experience in his head, thereby activating the network through reactivation of sensory systems. Such reliving can include guidance from the therapist to consider each sensory system, including touch and smell as well as vision and sound. Drawing can access the network through visual spatial means. Gestalt techniques that ask the client to assume various roles in the experience can access aspects of the network that could otherwise remain untouched by verbal discussion, since motor action is involved and since executive systems are focused on creating an experience rather than determining why. The client can be asked to notice the feelings involved or the experience as a whole with an admonition not to try to describe it in words, since the translation into words may interfere with more complete experience of the neural network. Use of the neural network concept thus supports use of an eclectic set of intervention techniques within a framework that guides selection of each technique when appropriate.

The neural network concept provides a framework within which clients' behaviors and expressions during therapy can be more effectively understood and treated. The concept supports identification of multiple contributors to a client's functioning, guides development of relevant interventions, and offers a language for including the client more actively in the therapy process. Within the context of neural networks various specific aspects of client functioning can be approached, including affect, anxiety, and memory. In addition, the neural network concept can support consideration of specific therapist processes during psychotherapy, as well as characteristics of client change over the course of treatment. Subsequent chapters address individual aspects of client functioning and psychotherapy process during treatment.

13

Affect in therapy

Emotions are particularly potent elements of neural networks. They have a central role in therapists' brain-based conceptualizations during therapy while also serving as a valuable focus during discussions with clients. Concepts related to emotions in personal functioning were outlined in Chapter 5. These concepts can be applied by clinicians throughout the process of therapy. The present chapter addresses how such applications unfold during therapy and emphasizes how such understanding can be shared with clients.

Clinical observations suggest that clients often feel threatened by the intensity, unpredictability, and uncontrollability of emotions. Clients often feel weak and inadequate simply because they are experiencing emotions, and they often sense that something is wrong with them for having strong emotional reactions. There seems to be a tendency for clients to perceive that emotions are synonymous with the self, and as a result, when emotions are negative or unacceptable, clients become convinced, or at least suspicious, that their inner core is unacceptable. Clients express particular distress when their emotions do not match the declaratively developed conscious value system to which the individual client adheres. The client experiences his inner self as being incongruent with what he wants his self to be.

Explicit discussion of the nature and likely evolutionary function of emotions can allow clients to accept emotions and then both use and manage them more effectively. Explaining the important role of emotions in the activation of neural networks seems particularly useful in such discussion. Emotions can be described to clients as facilitating encoding of important new information (McGaugh, 2004) while also serving as a primitive information processing system (LeDoux, 2002). Emotions can therefore be presented as important elements of normal day-to-day functioning. They can also be presented as part of an affect-based processing system that uses connections with sensory, integration, and motor areas in the brain to gather information directly from sensory systems, connect the new sensory experiences with past experiences that have previously generated similar emotions, and then send signals to motor systems in the brain to initiate action. This system can work completely independent of declarative memory systems involved in conscious decision making.

The characteristics of such a system can be illustrated in concrete ways that help the client to grasp the concept. For example, a fist coming toward one's face strikes fear and prompts sudden evasive action; if a person took time to consciously evaluate factors of strength, rate of speed, and the likelihood that the striker will hold back at the last minute, one would be guaranteed a bloody if not broken nose. At the same time, it can also be illustrated that emotions can be misguided. If a consequence of past abuse by an uncle with a beard is that the client is currently fearful around all men with beards, it is clear that the emotional reaction is a misleading assessment of current information when it is applied to a kindly colleague at work, or to Santa Claus.

Details of emotional processing can be specifically delineated as part of clinical conceptualization and discussion with the client. It appears information incorporated during the experience of emotion is gathered in a parallel rather than a linear way. Sensory cortices as well as polymodal sensory integration areas have direct projections to the amygdala (LeDoux, 1996), with information from various areas arriving almost simultaneously. Consistent with elements of the neural network concept (see Chapter 3), amygdala 'affect' neurons previously associated with a particular pattern of sensory input and brain activation will fire when that particular neural pattern occurs again. The resulting emotion may be the first part of the neural network that comes into consciousness; that is, the emotion seems to just pop into existence. This accounts for a common perception among clients that emotions are unexplainable. If a person begins to feel sad for no obvious reason, it is likely that experiences around the person have triggered sadness in ways of which the person is not aware. The emotion has popped into the person's head.

Emotions that pop into awareness have connections with motor neurons as part of the related neural network (Derryberry & Tucker, 1992). Emotions thus influence thinking and action directly, which helps explain the strong inclination clients have to act on their feelings. If someone feels sad, the person may want to withdraw from interactions with others even if the demands of the workplace require that the person be socially active at the moment. It can be explained to clients that people differ in how strongly they consciously believe they must act on emotions and in how strongly they feel unconsciously compelled to display emotions they experience.

Emotions communicate extremely valuable information regarding the client's previous experiences, but this information often fails to match the total reality of the current situation that triggered the emotion – even though there are similarities between current and past experience. Such a view of emotions can be explicitly presented to clients to help them begin to respond to emotions in a different way. The sadness a client experiences may be related to memories of past events that are triggered by something at work, but the sadness and the previous memories may not be relevant to the client's current work setting. Clients may then be encouraged to save the information for later processing. It is important to use frontal, declarative, conscious processing systems to help assess the emotion that has emerged, and then to decide how to include the emotion in the final decision to act. In this way, emotions can be an integral and valuable part of rational decision-making regarding current beliefs and actions.

A problem with emotions is that because they strongly influence higher cortical thinking as well as inclinations toward action, they can interfere with adaptive action, whether the person experiencing the emotions consciously wants to act on them or not. If a client is feeling sad at work she may misperceive others as being hurtful toward her because her perception is influenced by the sadness she is feeling. She will be likely to interpret incoming information as congruent with the sadness she is feeling. More broadly, the client may feel sadness whenever she does not have a very intimate relationship with the person with whom she is working. Such a pattern of emotional response may reflect an internal neural network that is strongly entrenched for both genetic reasons and reasons of past experience, and the pattern may therefore be difficult to alter and impossible to eliminate.

When emotions are counter to what a person wants to feel, or are counter to a person's value system, such incongruence is important to include in the conscious decision-making process. If the client is feeling so sad at the moment that she cannot behave appropriately in the workplace, it may be worthwhile for her to "call in sick" until she is able to return to her more typical adequate functioning. If she is feeling sad on a chronic basis because of an underlying need to be more intimate with people than the current work setting allows, the client may need to look for a different job, since the current job does not match her nature. That is, the client is inclined to think and act in accordance with the brain connections that have been established in the past, and it is natural and useful to consider such inclinations when she is making decisions regarding current activities in which to engage in life.

Various non-brain metaphors have been found useful in helping people understand and cope with emotions. Emotions can be viewed as waves at the beach. Surfers cope with waves by riding them, not by trying to stop them;

they derive enjoyment from an experience that would be overwhelming if they tried to stop it. Thus, people can best cope with emotions by seeing what the emotions have to say and viewing them as avenues toward personal gratification rather than as something to be stopped.

Emotions can also be viewed as a river. Dams are typically not built to stop a river, but to manage it. If one tries to stop a river with a dam, eventually the water overflows the dam and destroys it. Similarly, if people try to stop their emotions completely they often feel overwhelmed because emotions eventually leak out; increased feelings of loss of self-control are the result.

Avoidance of emotions may sometimes be successful in some ways, with the erection of a brick wall against emotions being the metaphor for such success. However, a brick wall is viewed as being indiscriminate: the wall blocks all emotions rather than just the negative ones a person would like to exclude. A successful brick wall against emotions leads to lack of positive emotions when doing things that are congruent with the nature of the person, and, as a result, life as a whole becomes non-gratifying. It also leads to lack of negative emotions, and therefore reduces a person's awareness that they are doing something that runs counter to valid implicit, affect laden memories of what has been gratifying and what has not.

A graphic metaphor illustrating the dangerous impact of eliminating negative emotions is to ask the client to imagine the effects of being able to eliminate the pain associated with placing one's hand on a hot stove; the hand would be destroyed. It becomes clear that pain, emotional or physical, has value. If positive and negative feelings are successfully blocked, clients are then likely to make choices that do not match the psychological, brain-based nature of the client, and are therefore likely to result in problems for the client.

During discussion of emotions it can be made clear that sensations are different from emotions (Basbaum & Jessell, 2000). Input from sensory systems can go directly to reward or pain centers in the brain without being processed through integration systems that connect new information with emotions involved with declarative or implicit memories of past experience. Sensations may become substitutes for emotions; substance abuse and thrill seeking become more important as sources of gratification when emotions have been cut off, blocked off behind a wall. Substance abuse, thrill seeking, and self-mutilation may also be used to distract the client from emotional pain within (Paris, 2005). In terms of the metaphor of the wall, these behaviors become part of the wall holding back emotions.

A caveat needs to be kept in mind when deciding how to help a client integrate emotions into the process of therapy. When there are indications of the presence of Borderline Personality Disorder, Bipolar Disorder, or predictable problems with emotional lability it is often more appropriate to focus on helping the client limit emotional reactivity rather than explore such activity in an unbridled way. If it becomes evident that the client is likely to become emotionally overwhelmed during exploration of connections between neural networks, it can be explained that it appears that the client's affect centers are so responsive that it will be helpful to limit the client's engagement with that aspect of her processing.

Such an explanation is one example of describing a psychological problem as resulting from maladaptive activity in a small area of the brain instead of conceiving of the client as a whole being out of control. Even though emotions are experienced as overwhelming at times, the recognition that one area of the brain is the source of the problem helps the client identify with the many other parts of the brain that are functioning appropriately. Referring to the diagram of areas of the brain involved in different brain functions (Figure 1.1) and to the Big Picture diagram (Figure 9.1) can graphically emphasize to the therapist and the client that many areas of adaptive functioning are present even when emotions are poorly modulated. Positive self-esteem is then easier to establish and maintain despite the presence of strong emotions. Neurally conceived, such an explanation begins to encourage activation of declarative, executive, frontal lobe connections simultaneously with the experience of being emotionally overwhelmed; connections between positive adaptation networks and networks related to the emotion can then be developed that help change the intensity of the emotion over time. The client can be told, "When you begin to feel emotionally overwhelmed, remind yourself that such emotionality is expected based on what we have been talking about, and in that way you can at least remember what is contributing to the emotion being so strong".

The identification of affect as overwhelming can guide the therapist to focus with the client on developing coping skills for handling emotions rather than trying to uncover and identify the feelings. Discussion of which elements of the Big Picture support which types of adaptive functioning can help identify more clearly the pathway toward better functioning. Referring to Figure 9.1, it can be explained that using Executive Function systems to choose to engage in learning relaxation skills may be an important precursor to exploring strong emotions. This calms Arousal systems that can contribute to the overwhelming intensity of the emotion. The psychodynamic concept of supporting the defense functions in this way. If the person has managed his emotions throughout his life by immersing himself in his work, it may be useful to practice consciously switching focus to work successes rather than focusing on emotions that are so strong the person feels inadequate and ineffectual to the point of behavioral paralysis. Through such refocusing, neural networks that do not include overwhelming emotion become activated, providing relief.

By practicing such refocusing, the client develops skills associated with shifting focus, feels less overwhelmed and intimidated by the experience of emotions, and begins to develop neural networks related to positive self-esteem.

Even dissociative strategies may be effective in removing a client from a potentially overwhelming emotional experience, and judicious use of such strategies may be adaptive even though unplanned dissociative events may be maladaptive. Neural networks not attached to the overwhelming emotion are activated by such strategies. If a client has overwhelming negative emotions in response to any sexual contact due to a history of abuse, it may be adaptive for the client to rely on dissociative disengagement during appropriate consensual sexual interactions. Marriages or other intimate relationships can be supported while the client works through the time consuming process of reworking neural networks tied to the previous abuse.

When emotional lability during a session appears likely to interfere substantially with the client's adaptive functioning, the therapist can alter the way in which related neural networks are explored. It may be important to switch the focus of therapy from emotion to intellectualization in order to preserve the client's capacity to continue working on the current therapeutic issue. Activating frontal lobe executive functions can compete with networks characterized by extreme emotion. The therapist can serve as a modulator of affect for the client when the client has difficulty modulating affect by himself. In such cases, rather than ask the client to notice the sensations and related feelings tied to problematic situations, the therapist can use intellectual descriptions and summaries of what has already been presented. When the concept of neural networks is explained, and when connections between previous experiences, emotions in general, and current experience are outlined in reference to neural systems involved, affect tends to fade because the intellectual explanations are novel and not likely to include in their neural networks so many direct connections with affect centers.

Observing the client's behavioral responses such as tears, flushing, or a panicky look in the eyes provides information regarding whether the neural network being triggered is far enough removed from affect to allow steady functioning. This permits the exploration of neural networks relevant to the issue at hand without an overwhelming affect disrupting the overall functioning of the brain. At a later time it may be possible to attach this newly constructed, declarative neural network to overwhelming emotions in such a way that the new but well-established network has a greater chance of modulating the affect.

Once it is decided that the level of emotionality experienced by the client is likely to be manageable, the concept of different types of memory systems can be used to guide working through the emotional material. When a client has identified a particular experiential history that accounts for the emotional lability, for example, early traumatic abuse, it can be pointed out that even though insight regarding the source is present, the slow changing procedural memory systems will continue for an extended period of time to trigger affect that the fast changing declarative memory systems recognize is not adaptive or appropriate in the current situation. The process of weakening those procedural memory links requires multiple rehearsals so that both declarative and procedural memory systems can develop links between more positive affect and the sensory patterns involved while also habituating the maladaptive connections previously established.

The client can also be reminded that the procedural memories supporting such maladaptive emotional responding are likely to have been reasonable responses to the situations the client experienced as a younger person. The client can therefore view the experience of overwhelming emotions as understandable rather than a sign the client is "crazy". The importance of replacing crazy with a reasonable explanation is that crazy implies both global dysfunction and impossibilities of being understood or managed. In contrast, identifying the maladaptive process as overwhelming but understandable allays those fears, allowing the client to deal solely with the emotion rather than the loss of organization of the whole realm of experience.

The model for understanding the overwhelming emotions also provides clear guides toward taking actions that are likely to positively influence the course of the previously imperturbable negative flow of affect. Neural networks related to self-efficacy can thus begin to be connected to the experience of powerful emotion. When the identified source of emotional explosiveness is best accounted for by genetic inclination, for example, because males throughout the family tree have experienced very strong emotional outbursts, explanations based on brain function can offer understanding and guidance as well. It can be explained that it is likely that genetically based wiring patterns contribute to an overactive emotion system; the person has an emotional on–off switch rather than a rheostat that gradually changes levels of emotional intensity. The client can be encouraged to observe triggers that likely set off emotional outbursts; these triggers are viewed as elements of neural networks that stimulate the affect centers to turn on explosively. It can be explained that such observations can lead to strategies for avoiding the triggering of such outbursts. At the same time, the client can be encouraged to identify and rehearse strategies for responding to the presence of intense internal emotions. For example, withdrawal to a private place, using a punching bag, or taking a walk can be reviewed as ways to diffuse the emotion. Rehearsing such strategies repeatedly, whether through imagery or role-play, makes it more likely that using such strategies will pop into the client's head when the emotions are occurring.

Intervening with medication is another strategy for managing emotions. Conceptualizing the role of medication within the brain–behavior paradigm emphasizes that medicine is going to help manage only a certain aspect of the functioning of the person's brain. This provides reassurance to the client that just because medicine is likely to be helpful, the whole self is not bad and the whole self will not be altered.

In addition to suggesting ways the interactions between various areas of the brain can be managed, a further implication of the concept of neural network for therapy is that the presence of the caring, calm, and understanding therapist during exploration of issues contributes to the development of modifications to maladaptive neural networks. These modifications are understood to compete with the negative affect that has interfered with functioning previously.

Some of the modifications conceived here are consistent with the concept of corrective emotional experience (Alexander & French, 1946) in that a specific past negative pattern of sensory experience associated with interpersonal relatedness is paired with a different, more adaptive tie between sensory experience and interpersonal relatedness. This pairing then allows for better functioning in the future. If relationships with all men have been bad in the past, but the client has a positive relationship with a male therapist, the sensory patterns representing men begin to be connected with positive emotions as part of the overall view of men. The changes are likely to occur in both declarative and procedural memory systems. If the client has always felt ineffectual in dealing with men, but now the client can voice opinions to the male therapist without experiencing devastating retaliation, senses of safety and self-efficacy become part of the networks representing relationships with men.

Some modifications to neural networks are conceived as different from the idea of corrective emotional experience based on change in the transferential relationship with the therapist. The presence of the calm therapist with whom the client feels secure helps develop a neural network that promotes calmness and security within the client when the client is meeting with the therapist. When this network is active at the same time that neural networks related to negative emotions are being actively explored in the session, a new sense of calmness begins to be associated with the experience of the problem. This is not viewed as a corrective emotional experience in which the therapy relationship and associated positive emotions begin to substitute for the previous relationship and past negative associations tied to that relationship. Rather, the emotions of feeling supported and secure help keep the client calm while confronting issues outside the relationship with the therapist, and senses of calmness and self-efficacy subsequently become attached to networks related to the problem. Consequently, the problem then does not feel so overwhelming. Positive emotions are added to the networks being explored rather than replacing the previous connections between sensory stimuli and the negative affect.

Neuroscience concepts allow emotions to be experienced and conceived as aspects of functioning that are part of the client rather than the core of the client, and neuroscience concepts then provide the basis for therapist and client to view emotions as identifiable aspects of the client that can be worked on and changed. This view encourages therapist and client to view emotions as resources rather than afflictions or weaknesses. Emotions can be perceived as supporting encoding and retrieval of memory rather than as primarily disrupting stable functioning. Emotions can be experienced as pathways to problem-resolution rather than solely problems to be managed. The unknowable nature of emotions can be better understood and accepted. It appears that adopting a neuroscience approach to emotions facilitates working with emotions during treatment while also empowering clients as people who can accept and cope with themselves in the course of daily life.

14

Memory and change

Many of the descriptions offered here regarding concepts related to neural networks and processing affect have included references to implicit and explicit memory processes. It is helpful to directly consider the implications of various aspects of memory during the process of therapeutic change.

Implicit memories are conceived as being based on simple connections between different neurons throughout the brain. The connections are strengthened slowly by multiple repetitions of connected neurons firing simultaneously (Kandel *et al.*, 2000b, pp. 1254–7). They weaken slowly through lack of simultaneous firing (Johnston, 2004; Kandel *et al.*, 2000b; Purves & Lichtman, 1985). One likely manner of weakening negative affect is through experiencing sensory stimuli while holding affect calm, thereby reducing the previous pairing of sensory (and other) neurons with negative emotions. Relaxation training combined with exposure during progressive desensitization (Wolpe, 1958) is a therapeutic intervention that achieves such a goal. Another likely manner of weakening is by way of habituation (Foa & Chambless, 1978; Kandel *et al.*, 2000b, pp. 1248–52); that is, the neuron pair is pressed, through exposure, to fire so often and for so long that neurotransmitters in the relevant synapses are temporarily used up, allowing the sensory (and other) neurons to fire without including simultaneous firing of affect neurons. Exposure with response prevention (Foa *et al.*, 1984) is an example of a psychotherapeutic intervention that achieves such a weakening. It should be noted that psychodynamic focus on issues could operate through the same mechanisms. That is, repeated exposure to issues in the therapy session could either pair calming with other neurons related to the issue at hand, or could expose the patient on an extended basis to the stimulus pattern so the relevant synapses go through the habituation process.

At the same time some synapses are weakening, other synapse pairs are likely to be strengthening. For example, while the person is habituating through exposure to neural network patterns that previously included distressing emotions, the person is also likely to be building a new network pattern that includes the same stimuli paired with benign or positive affect. Through implicit, procedural connections the person shifts their patterns of feeling and then behavior through the process of repeated exposure and processing. Various traditional psychotherapy intervention procedures activate these procedural processes, thereby leading to the first steps of change.

Implicit memories may be encoded without participation of hippocampal, declarative memory systems (Squire, 1992), or in addition to declarative encoding. Declarative encoding could be absent in memories of experiences that occurred before the age of 4 years old. If the child was repeatedly rebuffed by her depressed mother during the first 3 years of her life, then later sensitivity to rejection in intimate relationships could be an expression of such early, implicitly encoded rejection.

Declarative encoding could also be absent for aspects of memories that were below the threshold of awareness (Seitz & Watanabe, 2003). A person noticing the emotions associated with rejection might be encouraged to notice what pops into her head while experiencing such feelings. "I don't know why, but there is this image of my mother complimenting me . . . it feels bad . . . it's the tone . . . I remember not liking her compliments, but I never knew why". It could be that the tone was encoded but not consciously identified at the same time that declarative memory of the words of the compliments was encoded. In psychotherapy, it could be the healing process would include recognition of the negative tone, processing of reactions to the new declarative recognition, and exposure to compliments in the absence of the negative tone. This combination of processes would be expected to lead to habituation of the old connection while developing a new capacity for appreciating compliments.

LeDoux (1996) has suggested that the recovery of implicit memories, that is, bringing implicit memories into explicit awareness, may involve turning the implicit memory into a conscious memory for the first time. The processing of severe trauma offers a good example of this process. It is hypothesized that at the time the severe trauma occurred the hippocampus was deactivated by the high level of distress. Helping the trauma victim recover a memory of a traumatic event brings that memory into awareness for the first time.

This is not the same as uncovering a repressed memory whereby previously conscious memory is driven from awareness by means of psychodynamic defenses and then later recalled; rather, the traumatic memory was never encoded in declarative memory because of deactivation of the hippocampus. Clinical observations suggest that recall of previously implicit memories "starts the clock ticking" with regard to dealing with the event. It is as if the event has just occurred, and the steps of coping follow the grief recovery process as the new memory is integrated into the person's previously developed sense of self. For example, in working with a rape victim it is as if the person were raped at the time the memory was recovered, and begins the healing process with the recovery of that memory.

Memory researchers have raised questions regarding the veridicality of recovered implicit memories of trauma (Jacobs & Nadel, 1998). They have suggested that typical explicit memory processes and the processes associated with recovering implicit memories of traumatic events both involve retrieval of memory fragments, filling in gaps by means of inference, and fitting the fragments into a context so that they are then experienced as an explicit, autobiographical memory. The difference between the two types of events is that normal autobiographical memories have been encoded using the context supplied by explicit hippocampal memory processes, while traumatic memories have been stored without benefit of or connection to the explicit contextual memory system. Researchers exploring the development of false memories have identified multiple ways in which benign memories can be distorted during encoding and retrieval (Loftus & Hoffman, 1989; Okado & Stark, 2005), and it seems likely that recovered memories of trauma would be influenced by such processes as much or more than would benign memories since the tie to an encoding context is lacking. This research suggests that clinicians working with clients who report such memories of trauma must consciously avoid influencing the abuse victim toward believing specific facts about the abuse experience since the lack of an encoding context could leave the client highly vulnerable to being influenced by external input.

It appears that research into false memories does not call into question the existence of memory processes that could maintain implicit traumatic memories. In fact, recent neuroimaging research offers support for the existence of flashbacks that are not connected to explicit memory processes (Lanius *et al.*, 2004). Instead, research into false memories highlights the vulnerability of any memory to distortion, and suggests that when working with victims reporting abuse the clinician should consciously avoid activities that could provoke creation of new details during the process of recovery.

The process of recovering, or discovering, implicit memories leads to new connections being attached to the old implicit patterns. It is expected that these new connections can support positive adaptive functioning in the future. As conceived in the present model, connecting explicit awareness with the implicit memory pattern makes it more likely that when the implicit pattern occurs in the future, the newly associated explicit memory will also be triggered. The person can then add thoughtful consideration to the previously unconscious pattern of responding. The inclusion of understanding and acceptance of the maladaptive response pattern can reduce the severity of the negative reaction while the person can also choose to make different choices. If the person is afraid to enter social settings because of an underlying, previously unconscious, wish to avoid the sadness of not being accepted, the person can choose to enter social situations anyway, thereby supporting the development of a history of social success that competes with the old, maladaptive expectations of failure. If the person experiencing panic at the initiation of intimacy realizes the panic is associated with previous abuse, the person can begin to develop awareness that the neural network associated with current appropriate intimacy is very different from neural networks associated with earlier trauma, even though some of the same sensations and responses are included in each network.

Explicit memory processes are conceived to operate quite differently than implicit ones. A better understanding of these differences can lead to better understanding of how explicit and implicit memory systems interact to support change in psychotherapy. The hippocampus is a primary center for long term potentiation, a form of learning that supports establishing new connections between several cells (Kandel, 2000) (see Figure 4.1). The process is a modification of the basic bi-cellular process that appears to be the foundation of procedural, implicit memory throughout the rest of the brain. The high level of occurrence of long-term potentiation within the hippocampus helps explain its unique role in supporting rapid acquisition of new information, of which novel insight during therapy is an example.

Some details of long-term potentiation were described in the earlier chapter on memory (Chapter 4). Long-term potentiation provides a model for considering how two previously unconnected cells can begin to trigger the same response; it is a model of how novel learning can occur. The intercellular model of long-term potentiation suggests simultaneously bringing into a client's consciousness two competing concepts, thereby increasing the connections between them. An example of this could be the previously described experience of a man with a beard triggering fear because of past abuse experiences. If the client is helped to relax before confronting the image of the past perpetrator, then when the image is brought to mind, the firing of calm signals will also be paired with the image, and the calm signals will then more likely be associated with images of bearded men in the future. A novel connection has been established. It may take multiple exposures in order for the negative emotional experience to habituate and the connection with calmness to become stronger, but establishing connections between the image and the new emotional network initiates a change.

The hippocampus is particularly well suited for such learning because of the presence of layers densely packed with pyramidal cells (Schwartz & Westbrook, 2000). These cells have large numbers of dendrites bringing in information from all over the brain. As demonstrated in Figure 4.2, the hippocampus is well situated to receive this information. The pyramidal cells are also highly interconnected with each other. Hippocampal pyramidal cells thereby support the development of new connections between input from different parts of the brain through these multiple connections and the long-term potentiation process. This process of integrating information from diverse parts of the brain supports integration of executive decision-making processes based in the frontal lobes with sensory experience, affect, and procedural types of integration in other parts of the brain. Within the present model this integration is understood to support the integration of declarative memory processes with procedural ones.

One aspect of psychotherapy appears to involve the activation of implicit memories while explicit memory systems are functioning, thereby making previously unconscious implicit memories available to declarative processing. Research has shown that as part of conscious, declarative functioning the frontal lobes serve the role of enhancing the processing of information in other parts of the brain through priming and similar processes (Posner & Raichle, 1994). The frontal lobes are also understood to offer inhibitory, stop-and-think mechanisms that can delay expression while explicit processing is completed (Casey et al., 2000). Establishing neural connections between explicit and implicit memories is viewed as enhancing the power of the frontal lobes to influence implicit memories. Because executive decision-making in the frontal lobes is viewed as supporting conscious, adaptive use of perceptions and memories, this increases the likelihood the client will begin to adaptively manage past memories rather than blindly act out the motor elements of previously established implicit neural networks.

The previously used example of the client previously abused by the bearded man can help understand the unfolding of connections between implicit and explicit memories. In the example, a client was abused as a child by an uncle with a beard. As a result, because of shared neurons in the two neural networks, an affectively neutral man with a beard encountered later in life evokes the network associated with previous abuse by a man with a beard. Negative emotions that previously occurred during the abuse are then elicited. When, with the help of the supportive, calming therapist, the client becomes aware of the ties between the two experiences, new connections between frontal decision-making processes and the implicit, previously learned network are established. It is then likely that when the implicit memory is triggered, thoughts and ideas that are part of frontal decision-making are also activated. Rationality and irrationality occur simultaneously. At this point the client has a better understanding of why the given emotions are occurring, even though the person may not be able to control these emotions. Repeated experience of this process will more firmly establish the connection between rational consideration and the maladaptive emotions experienced by the client.

A critical implication of this model of change is that inclusion of the frontal lobes in neural networks initially composed of implicit connections between sensory experience, affect, and motor neurons is not expected to suddenly eliminate the maladaptive responses triggered by the implicit memories involved. In fact, because the connections between sensory/affect experiences and motor centers are likely to remain strong since procedural neural connections change slowly, a person is likely to act on the maladaptive implicit memories even though the person "knows better".

The abused client described earlier may understand that his emotional reactions to the man with the beard are irrational, maladaptive reactions based on earlier abuse by an uncle who had a beard, but he may still experience such intense reactions that the client chooses to endure other hardships rather than be in the same room with the current, benign bearded male.

A different client may recognize that sadness experienced during arguments with a spouse is unreasonably strong because of an early history of her parents becoming emotionally withdrawn whenever she disappointed them. However, the current sadness may still result in the client spending days in bed after arguments with her spouse because of the intensity of feelings of loss – even though there is no indication that divorce will occur.

Often clients interpret the inability of insight to immediately alter a previously established maladaptive pattern of behavior as indicating the client is permanently defective. Therapists are at risk for making the same assumption about the client. Maintaining a view that procedural memories require multiple repetitions in order for change to occur allows therapist and client to accept the slowness of change in therapy without giving up hope. It also helps them to remain focused on taking steps that are likely to lead to improvement even though incongruity between cognitive under-standing and behavioral or emotional responsiveness may be present.

It is understood in the present conceptualization that change during psychotherapy often requires the concurrent presence of old, maladaptive neural networks and new adaptive networks. It is also assumed that the old pattern will not be reinforced by the current environment, and therefore the neural connections that support unrealistic aspects of the network will become weaker. It is also assumed that newer, more adaptive connections will become more solidly connected with elements of the older neural network so that eventually a newer, more adaptive network becomes strong enough to become the primary influence on emotion and behavior. After a clear understanding, based in declarative memory processes, of an emotional situation is established, the client is encouraged to experience related situations while maintaining awareness of the incongruity between the disparate adaptive and maladaptive reactions to the situation. It is understood, and stated explicitly, that the client may continue to respond maladaptively in various ways even while recognizing the responses are maladaptive. At the same time, it is assumed that the simultaneous occurrence of adaptive and maladaptive views will lead to weakening of the maladaptive view while the adaptive view is strengthening, resulting in eventual change.

Cognitive behavioral theorists have discussed the necessity of having a complete "schema" included in therapeutic work in order for change to occur (Lang, 1979). The current model fits with this admonition. If an important aspect of the maladaptive experience is not identified in the course of exploring the thoughts, images, and feelings involved, then when adaptive neural networks are included in the experience, the simultaneous processes of habituation and development of adaptive neural connections with previous experiences will not occur completely. The unidentified element of the maladaptive neural network may continue to trigger negative emotions and behaviors in unexplained ways, leading to demoralization in the client.

For example, if a history of sexual abuse of a client included some elements of pleasure despite the predominant elements of pain and fear, then simultaneous experience of current positive, appropriate sexual behavior in the presence of past expectations of fear and pain will not eliminate irrational reactions during the current sexual contact. This is likely no matter how often the client rehearses the experience. The connections between pleasure and the sexual event will not be shifting during re-experience. It is probably necessary for the client to recognize the presence of pleasure in the previous events, work through the shame involved, and then repeat current sexual experiences while recognizing that shame will be an automatic response whenever pleasure occurs. Appropriate shifting in the connections between the current and past neural networks is then more likely to occur.

The process of identifying the maladaptive neural network in the presence of declarative memory processes has implications for under-standing the concept of repression. Identification of previously established maladaptive networks likely involves both uncovering and discovering processes. Uncovering seems synonymous with the psychodynamic process of exposing repressed memories while working through defenses (Fenichel, 1945). Early negative experiences of which the client was originally aware come to elicit anxiety whenever the brain's monitoring systems identify a neural pattern as being too similar to the previous negative experience. Defensive procedures are then activated, reducing the likelihood of the unacceptable pattern continuing to unfold. This process prevents conscious awareness of the source of distress while activating defensive behaviors such as working too hard, engaging in substance abuse, or initiating aggressive interactions with people so that power rather than weakness is activated. Identifying the maladaptive nature of the defensive procedures, recognizing the anxiety, allowing thoughts to pop into awareness, and then exploring them more fully can lead to undoing of the repression and working through the establishment of more adaptive responses as outlined above.

Discovering, however, involves establishing connections between declarative memory and elements of procedural memory of which the client has never been aware (LeDoux, 1996). Processing of flashbacks provides the clearest example of such work. The traumatic experience, for example, of a fire-fight in Vietnam, is assumed to have been so emotionally powerful that hippocampal, long-term memory processes were disrupted to such a degree that a declarative memory was never established. However, connections between the amygdala and various sensory and motor systems are assumed to have remained active at a high level during the traumatic experience. Working through the flashback involves the process of the declarative memory systems discovering what was never consciously recorded, that is, was never recorded in declarative memory.

The encoding of trauma is an extreme example of declarative memory processes not being involved in establishing a memory of an event. There is evidence, as well, that elements of non-traumatic experience are encoded without the involvement of the hippocampus and long-term memory processes (Seitz & Watanabe, 2003). It is assumed such encoding occurs throughout day-to-day functioning. It therefore seems likely that during the establishment of maladaptive patterns, declarative and procedural memories are simultaneously being established, both of which will influence future behavior. In the current view some of these procedural memories are unconscious because they were not declaratively recorded rather than because they were repressed. The current model also suggests that some aspects of an experience may be connected to declarative memory, while other aspects of the same experience may not be connected to declarative memory. For example, a war veteran might have explicit memories of the initial events during a fire-fight, but have only implicit memories after a particularly horrible occurrence during the fight. The line between uncovering and discovering procedural memories becomes fuzzy in such situations.

The process of the hippocampus shutting down during high stress may be viewed to be one way the brain protects itself, and may therefore be viewed as a defensive procedure. However, the processes of repressing an aware memory and failing to declaratively encode a traumatic one seem different enough to warrant different understanding and different interventions. Recovery from a repressed memory would require working through defenses that have developed to manage anxiety over an extended period. In addition, anxiety triggered by newly discovering a traumatic memory never encoded in declarative systems might have fewer entrenched defenses blocking exploration.

It is also possible that a procedural memory of childhood abuse could include elements that are threatening to the adult beginning to recall the trauma, but were not threatening when the client was experiencing the abuse as a child. For example, it is possible that a person sexually abused as a small child did not experience shame during the abuse. This could happen if the victim was too young to understand shame. However, if the person was later taught that sexuality is shameful, then if procedural memories of sexual abuse began to emerge into awareness, shame networks would be triggered that were not part of the original traumatic abuse experience. These shame networks not originally connected to the abuse would then be expected to trigger anxiety. It is assumed that shame in this example would not be intensely connected to networks associated with the trauma of abuse, and it is assumed the connections with fear, pain, and anxiety would be less intense. It would still be necessary to confront issues related to shame, but the intensity of such work would probably be lower, and the rate of change would likely be faster.

Connecting declarative memory systems to previously established maladaptive procedural memories is important in several ways. As described in Chapter 6, Gray (1982) offered a model of anxiety in which experiences can elicit anxiety if they have previously been connected to aversive stimuli or if they are novel. The contribution of novelty is likely to begin to dissipate if the client understands the nature of the past neural network being activated. This can reduce the negative emotional experience associated with such recall.

Conscious, declarative understanding of newly recognized painful procedural memories can help the client endure the negative emotions associated with awareness of previous negative experiences. This under-standing can support the client while the client is developing new adaptive responses even though these new patterns temporarily activate emotional pain associated with negative past experiences.

Conscious processes can include frontal lobe executive functioning that helps inhibit negative behaviors that have been part of previous maladaptive neural networks. Frontal executive functioning can also help activate new ways of coping with internal feelings and external events.

Furthermore, it is also possible that when the client intentionally confronts past memories, underlying neural substrates supporting activity rather than substrates supporting passivity (see Derryberry & Tucker, 1992) become connected to the previous maladaptive neural network, thereby helping the client replace helplessness with effectiveness.

Finally, the slowness of change in procedural connections has the potential to result in the client giving up when change is not quickly forthcoming. Awareness of how declarative systems can influence procedural systems can offer encouragement and structure that support continuing participation in activities likely to lead to positive change in the long run. Thus, while establishing new connections between declarative memory processes and the old procedural memory is not likely to immediately eliminate maladaptive emotional responses or behaviors, engaging the declarative processing systems offers multiple ways to begin to effectively facilitate positive change.

Reflecting on the processes of habituation and sensitization (Kandel et al., 2000b) in procedural memory highlights a potential problem in dealing with negative affect-laden memories. Part of the rationale for exposing the client to previous negative emotional experiences is that such exposure can lead to habituation to the memory. Repeated, prolonged exposure is assumed to lead to reduced activity in related neural connections. However, it seems theoretically possible that rather than habituating to the exposure, the repeated exposures could actually be sensitizing the person to the negative experience. In addition, the possible re-traumatization of the client during such exposures could contribute to further impairment in hippocampal functioning, leading to harm being done to the client. The question is difficult to resolve because the hypothesized need for repeated exposure during the process of habituation assumes that severe emotional reaction will continue to occur for an extended period of time even though improvement is occurring.

The current approach suggested for dealing with this conundrum includes recognition that successful exposure treatment techniques for traumatized rape victims involve high levels of affective response but have still yielded positive results (Foa et al., 1991). Furthermore, there is evidence with clients suffering from obsessive-compulsive disorder that gradual exposure is as effective as flooding the client with the full negative experience (Boersma et al., 1976). These studies suggest exposure to negative memories is useful, and that less rapid and therefore less intense emotional exposure techniques may be appropriate.

It is suggested that applying exposure techniques should include comparing the relative potential negative impacts of leaving the current maladaptive patterns unchanged with the potential negative impacts of experiencing sensitization to the experience through attempts at exposure. If the probable negative impact of the historical maladaptive pattern is high, then the potential relative risk associated with exposure may be warranted.

Such decisions can be discussed with the client, thereby developing informed consent for participation in the exposure while also helping the client experience her own processes as understandable and therefore less overwhelming even when strong emotion and inappropriate actions remain.

Memory can be considered in reference to the Big Picture model even though there is no specific reference to memory in the outline of the model. Explicit and implicit memories can be examined with regard to what influences the various elements of the model have on the neural networks involved in the memories. For example, an implicit memory developed without involvement of hippocampus and frontal lobes because of the trauma involved would be viewed as not connected to Frontal Executive systems. A client with weak verbal processing would be expected to have memories that emphasize non-verbal brain centers represented within the Integration systems in the top row of Figure 9.1. Different memories will involve Arousal, Emotion, Anxiety, and past Patterns of experience to different degrees, and the framework of the Big Picture model can guide consideration of how memory systems interact in the expression of the client's difficulties.

In summary, consideration of change in relation to implicit and explicit memory systems adds to the understanding and implementation of change in clients. It is clear that change is likely to occur at multiple levels of awareness and multiple levels of brain function. Implicit memories will require multiple exposures over an extended period of time in order for change to be achieved. Explicit memory systems are likely to change more rapidly, with the classical experience of insight demonstrating the speed of such change. Changes in explicit and implicit systems are likely not to be synchronous, which can be disconcerting to clients and therapists hoping for change, but which is also the basis for using explicit systems to support change in implicit systems. Interactions between explicit and implicit systems suggest the intervention of having the client maintain awareness of differences between the two systems rather than encouraging the client to work aggressively to change the implicit system, since the implicit system is expected to change slowly no matter how intensively the person tries to make the neural network change. Understanding the two memory systems thus helps facilitate change while also helping maintain calm and acceptance while going through the change process.

15

Anxiety and change

The roles of anxiety in the change process warrant special consideration. The basic relationship of anxiety to the overall model of brain function and psychotherapy has been previously discussed (see Figure 6.1), so only a brief summary is presented here. Gray has posited the presence of a system that monitors the similarity between brain patterns related to current experience and brain patterns that have been associated with negative events in the past. When the system identifies similarity, the anxiety response is triggered. This involves behavioral inhibition, increased diffuse arousal, and increased attention to the environment. Anxiety itself likely blocks awareness of the source of the anxiety through diffuse brain arousal that interferes with a particular pattern standing out from other patterns and therefore gaining attention. Behaviors that reduce the similarity between current patterns and past distressing patterns likely reduce the anxiety reaction, and in this way maladaptive behaviors that avoid dealing with a problem are rewarded. These maladaptive patterns of experience and function present in therapy as anxiety that occurs for no obvious reason followed by behaviors that interfere with positive functioning.

When therapy reaches a road block whereby reasons for the anxiety and maladaptive behaviors are unclear, it becomes useful to recall that the anxiety response is part of a neural network. Previously discussed strategies for exploring neural networks can then be applied. The relationship of anxiety to the neural network is outlined to the client so that the client has a rationale for engaging in behaviors that increase rather than decrease stress in the short term. It can be explained that anxiety is often a response to negative feelings or situations, that the anxiety response blocks awareness of negative feelings, and that it is likely that current anxiety is blocking understanding of what the client's brain is experiencing at the moment. The client is then encouraged to "move toward the anxiety." That is, the client is encouraged to experience the sense of anxiety and notice what pops into the client's head. Such a strategy can be used with clients experiencing problems identified as anxiety disorders, such as Generalized Anxiety Disorder and Panic Disorder, as well as with clients who begin experiencing anxiety as part of another disorder, such as depression, or with clients who experience anxiety in only specific situations.

An example can demonstrate the process of following the anxiety. A mildly depressed client might present with difficulty maintaining motivation during completion of tasks in the home even though the tasks are chosen by the client. It would be useful to explore neural networks associated with difficulty completing a preferred task. The client could be asked to imagine initiating and then completing a specific task. This would activate relevant neural networks. If signs of anxiety developed, the therapist could ask the client to notice the anxiety and then notice what pops into his head. It is likely that a string of images would be presented, and it is also likely that an image would be described that ties anxiety to another distressing situation. The client might report an image of completing chores at home alone as a child, and might then report sadness. The client might then shift back to thinking about the task he originally tried to imagine. The series of thoughts just described flows from identification of the problem to imagining the problem situation to experiencing anxiety to noticing other cognitions to noticing feelings and finally back to the original problem. In this case, following anxiety guided the therapy to focusing on feeling abandoned while completing tasks.

When anxiety is addressed as part of the neural network it often serves as the red flag that guides the client and therapist toward resolution of the problem. "When we are lost in therapy, move toward the guiding flag of anxiety", is an instruction that can be specifically expressed to the client. The client is encouraged to identify the presence of anxiety when it occurs. Even though the anxiety does not make obvious sense at the moment that it is first noticed, it is assumed that it is information that can be understood if the client takes time to attend to it.

The client is helped to allow the related neural network to become more active. This can be done in ways that are typically used to activate a network more fully. The client is encouraged to notice thoughts, visual images, sounds, and internal sensations that pop into the client's head as the sensation of anxiety is focused upon. In particular, the client is encouraged to notice and accept emotions that may begin to emerge. Almost by definition, such emotions are likely to be uncomfortable since the theory states that the anxiety is a reaction to the presence of something that is uncomfortable for the client. The relationship between anxiety and emotions can be specifically described for the client in order to help the client be familiar with and more accepting of the experiences they may have while following the connections between anxiety and the rest of the neural network. Often the process that began with following anxiety shifts to following the emotions that are subsequently identified, since emotions are likely to be more directly related to the issues that are causing the client's distress. At that point, guidelines outlined in previous discussions of exploring the neural network become relevant (see Chapter 12).

Gray suggested that novelty can serve as a trigger for anxiety (see Chapter 6). This connection can specifically guide understanding and interventions during the later stages of psychotherapy. When the therapist recognizes that the client is moving past previously maladaptive coping patterns toward newer, more adaptive functioning, the therapist can warn the client that anxiety can develop simply because the experience of functioning well is novel. For example, if a client was recovering from long-standing fear of rejection, she might begin to think of attending a social function and then find herself feeling anxious. If the fear of rejection is well-resolved, the therapist and client could discuss the possibility that the anxiety is occurring because the social setting is unfamiliar rather than because the client fears rejection. The difference between approaching a previously negative situation and approaching a novel situation can be outlined so that the client feels as familiar as possible with reactions she is likely to experience during upcoming events. Such a discussion provides new declarative memory connections with the upcoming novel event and the potential anxiety. As a result, the experience of the new event is actually more familiar and therefore less likely to trigger anxiety associated with novelty.

Clinical experience suggests that a primary way that the connection between novelty and anxiety is expressed is through the experience of "The Empty Head". As the client begins to let go of old, maladaptive patterns of functioning during therapy, the old emotional reactions become less powerful, increased awareness becomes part of the neural networks previously associated with pain and distress, and the client is ready to move on to new, more adaptive functioning. The neural network model suggests that as the client moves toward the new experiences, suddenly there will be a paucity of neural network connections. The paucity of neural connections appears to be one way in which novelty is expressed. If a female client has felt chronically inadequate and has spent many years establishing relationships by talking with others about her inadequacy, the client is likely to experience The Empty Head if she begins to feel satisfied with who she is. She will not know what to say, how to act, how to interpret incoming information, or even how to feel as an independent, self-assured woman because neural networks associated with positive self-esteem do not yet exist. The client does not have neural networks available for understanding or coping with interpersonal interactions. The emotions tying together procedural and decision-making systems have shifted toward being more positive (see Chapter 14).

It is assumed that emotions are a critical element in the neural network, particularly in activating sensory and motor procedural memory systems in a direct, intuitive way. Therefore, the positive emotion in a new situation will not be connected to sensory, motor, or integration elements of the neural network. As clients progress into the realm of new, positive functioning they may suddenly feel lost in a profound way that can easily trigger anxiety if not panic. The sense of becoming nothing is likely to feel intense, and possibly overwhelming. Visceral experiences such as dizziness and disorientation are likely to accompany more traditional symptoms of anxiety such as rapid heart rate, perspiration, and shallow breathing, among others.

The client experiencing the intense anxiety that can accompany the novelty of improvement is likely to believe that no progress has really been made. The client may think that progress has been poorly established and that the client has regressed to previous maladaptive ways of functioning. At this point the therapist's interpretation that the reaction is part of the nature of progress can provide reassurance, particularly if a strong working relationship has been previously established. Feelings of warmth and support accompanied by cognitive understanding of the phenomena of anxiety and The Empty Head can be associated with networks developing during this stage of change. This can reduce unfamiliarity as well as other feelings, such as loneliness, abandonment, and disorientation.

16

The experience of improvement in psychotherapy

Anxiety often offers the initial signal that neural networks are operating in unrecognized ways to disrupt the client's functioning. Anxiety often then guides the exploration of the network. In the case of anxiety related to the novelty intrinsic to psychological change, anxiety then signals the shift from processing past learning to creating a new future.

The next step implied by the description of novelty, anxiety, and The Empty Head is the facilitation of new neural connections in new, adaptive neural networks. Throughout discussion of neural networks and the activation of maladaptive functioning the importance of connecting adaptive networks to maladaptive ones has been emphasized. This process provides the basis for developing adaptive behaviors for the future. As the client confronts the sense of feeling lost that often accompanies change, networks associated with a history in therapy of confronting distress with the support of the therapist should be available to be activated. Such patterns compete with the sense of being lost and disoriented, reducing the intensity of such feelings. The client's relationship with the therapist accompanied by experiences of successfully coping with distress within the context of therapy can offer initial new networks with which to fill The Empty Head.

At this point in therapy the client needs to begin to develop neural patterns associated with positive coping, and these patterns need to be firmly connected to stimuli that previously triggered strong negative emotions, anxiety, and defensive behaviors that previously undermined successful adaptation to life. The therapist may need to help the client apply the client's own previously developed adaptive coping strategies during the resolution of problems currently being addressed in therapy. With regard to the brain, it is conceived that frontal executive systems are being planfully stimulated to foster the establishment of connections between neural patterns underlying coping and neural patterns that previously triggered maladaptive processes. A person who has displayed excellent planning and problem-solving in the work setting would be encouraged to apply such skills systematically toward increasing the amounts of appropriate physical intimacy with people at varying levels of relationship with the client. It is assumed that with repetition such connections would become more established and more likely to fire when the previously distress-invoking stimuli occur.

The therapist may need to help the client learn a totally new set of skills; that is, new neural networks may need to be intentionally developed. This is contrary to a classic psychodynamic approach in which the passive therapist allows but also requires the client to generate new coping patterns out of personal history. Social skills training (Bellak, 2004; Mersch et al., 1991) would be important for a person whose distress and anxiety have interfered with ongoing social interactions for many years. The person might need to be taught how to use open questions rather than closed questions during conversations, and might need to learn active listening skills that include summarizing what the other person has said. Non-verbal skills such as eye-contact and appropriate social distance may need to be taught. The client may need active, direct training in identifying internal feeling states and then expressing them in assertive rather than aggressive ways (Rakos, 1991). The client may need to learn relaxation skills in order to provide self-soothing when anger, anxiety, or sadness is experienced (Deffenbacher et al., 2002).

Throughout the teaching of such new skills the therapist should be alert for opportunities to hook up previously learned skills with the new ones being learned so that The Empty Head is filled in as quickly as possible, thereby reducing anxiety associated with change while simultaneously accessing more elaborate and well-entrenched patterns of coping. It is assumed that neural networks with a longer history of firing together will be more easily activated in the future and will be more resistant to disruption than will networks that are newer and have been repeated less often. Therefore, relying on older, previously adaptive coping networks when possible is advised. Such a consideration would suggest to a behavior therapist helping a client learn new appropriate behaviors to adapt a skills training module to include strengths idiosyncratic to the client rather than expect the client to rely solely and rigidly on the patterns suggested by the module.

Strengthening new neural connections that support adaptive behaviors does not appear to eliminate old connections. The assumption is that old connections are weakened through habituation and that new connections are strengthened in ways that compete with the weakening maladaptive connections of the past. Multiple repetitions of positive coping will slowly strengthen connections in related neural networks, and as a result these connections will be more likely to be triggered in the presence of previously negative stimuli. However, there are indications that residual effects of earlier negative experiences will not be eliminated. It has been proposed that sensitization and kindling processes emanating from stressful experiences result in a person being more susceptible to future psychological difficulties following the experiences of early stress or trauma (Breslau *et al.*, 1999; Post, 1992). It is therefore likely that the occurrence of either a previously experienced or a novel type of traumatic event will reactivate old response patterns in a sudden and powerful way. Research into trauma experienced by adults has indicated that people who have experienced trauma earlier in their lives are more likely to be traumatized by negative events later in life (Breslau *et al.*, 1999). Soldiers experiencing symptoms of Post Traumatic Stress Disorder (PTSD) are more likely to report having experienced childhood trauma than are soldiers who have not been identified with symptoms of PTSD (Bremner *et al.*, 1993). If clients are warned ahead of time about the possibility of such eruptions of past patterns during future events, and if they are provided rationales and strategies for dealing with such eruptions, it seems likely that they will not be as overwhelmed by their experience of the eruption, will not judge themselves so negatively, and will have greater capacity to cope effectively with the events when they occur.

In the present view what could be labeled regression is less pejoratively identified as a natural but unpleasant part of the process of life. It therefore does not need to be viewed as failure; rather it can be viewed as a reasonable and understandable part of the process of improvement that continues over the lifespan. Clients typically do not like hearing that such events may occur, but the benefit of understanding and being prepared to cope with such events appears to outweigh the distress of learning about the possibility.

The Big Picture model offers a concrete framework within which improvement can be considered. For example, as improvement unfolds it is likely relative activity levels in different areas of functioning will be observed to shift. If emotional dyscontrol was initially identified as a problem area, as therapy approaches its conclusion it is likely that either emotional volatility will have decreased, or executive function planning and inhibition processes will be working to manage the remaining volatility more effectively. If an area of integration has been identified as weak during the course of therapy, plans for functioning will have been developed either within the integration realm or outside the realm of integration whereby the negative effects of the integration deficit are reduced. For example, if verbal integration has been identified as a problem, resolution at the end of therapy may include relying on external prompts and reminders in order to carry out verbally based tasks, or resolution may include working at a job that does not require verbal integration. Therapeutic resolutions may include correction of the source of the problem, strategies for working around the problem, or elements of each. These are just two examples of how application of the Big Picture model can guide both therapist and client in considering how improvement has unfolded and whether enough change has occurred.

Consideration of brain functioning shapes understanding of improvement during psychotherapy and decisions regarding conclusion of treatment. Feelings of disorientation and distress are expected near the end of treatment when clients and therapists alike may expect feelings of increasing security and self-esteem. When it appears psychological problems are resolving adequately in therapy, neuroscience suggests the importance of actively helping the client develop new strategies for dealing with old situations. Finally, research regarding neuroscience suggests that realistic expectations for improvement include the possibility that there may be recurrences of problematic patterns, and preparing a client to expect and deal with these may enhance the stability of improvement in the long run.

17

The therapist's neuroscience

Chapters 12 to 16 examined aspects of clients' intrapsychic functioning and overt expression and behavior during psychotherapy in light of brain processes involved. At the same time that neuroscience concepts guide consideration of the client's processing and how to improve this processing, they can also guide understanding and use of the therapist's own brain functioning during therapy. The current chapter does not thoroughly explore the implications of neuroscience conceptualizations for therapist functioning. Rather, this chapter highlights some basic relevant implications that have been observed during the clinical process. General connections between neuroscience concepts and the therapist's functioning are described, the influences of the therapist's neural networks are outlined, limitations to reliance on intuition are identified, and ways to discuss with the client the therapist's neural networks are suggested. This chapter also addresses the implications for the client of the act of discussing the therapist's networks, describes the role of metaphor in the interaction between the client's and the therapist's neural networks, and highlights the importance of the therapist understanding as well as possible underlying patterns within the therapist that may shape the emergence of ideas and hunches into the therapist's conscious awareness.

A therapist's experiences during psychotherapy can be considered in light of all the aspects of neuroscience previously described in regard to client functioning. The therapist's functioning during therapy can be considered in light of the characteristics of input absorbed by the therapist, processing of information taken in, and outputs subsequent to this processing. In the course of the therapist's processing during interaction with a client all the different elements of The Big Picture (Figure 9.1) will contribute to and influence the therapist. Arousal systems, emotional processes, anxiety, neural networks, and executive functioning will all be part of brain activity within the therapist during therapy. Sensory images, increasing and decreasing arousal levels, shifting emotions, fluctuating anxiety, and both implicit and explicit memories within the therapist will all be based on the therapist's brain activity during treatment. Patterns of responses consisting of multiple neural networks will unfold in the therapist's brain during and across sessions. These patterns activated within the therapist during therapy will include networks associated with memories of earlier interactions with the client as well as with memories of the therapist's own past.

The overarching concept of neural networks incorporates the various elements of functioning within the therapist's brain. The therapist can actively tap the information held in his neural networks by noticing what "pops into his head". At the input stage of the therapist's input–process–output system, the therapist may take in information from the client without the therapist being consciously aware of such input. This information can trigger reactions in the therapist, such as specific emotions, for which the therapist cannot consciously account. In addition, information consciously taken in through explicit memory and learning systems may trigger both conscious explicit and unconscious implicit activity within the therapist's brain. It is assumed the therapist's consciously held understanding will be processed within the framework of the therapist's current awareness and his consciously-held therapeutic frame-work. However, it is also worthwhile for the therapist, upon encountering unexplained emotions, thoughts, or images, to consider that the cues coming from the client may be triggering the therapist's responses in unexpected and unacknowledged ways, and the responses are therefore worth using to guide therapy interventions.

The internal response within the therapist to such unexplained thoughts could be as simple as thinking to himself, "I don't know why, but I suddenly started feeling sad, and sometimes when that happens my response is related to something the client is experiencing". The therapist may suddenly recall something the client has said in the past. The client's description of the pain of losing a girlfriend may trigger recall by the therapist of the client's statement in an earlier session regarding his response to his parents' divorce. The therapist may immediately have a clear sense of the nature of the connection between the two statements by the client, or the therapist may not understand the connection. In either case, the sudden occurrence of the thought is conceived as an expression of the working of the therapist's neural networks tying experiences together and then prodding ideas into activation at a conscious level. The therapist will be using more of his own brain function in the therapeutic work if he can accept such emerging thoughts and feelings as valid and useable.

Thoughts that pop into the therapist's head may go beyond tying together elements in therapy of which the therapist has previously been aware. Theodore Reik, in his book, *Listening with the Third Ear*, described a situation in which, while listening to a female client, he noticed a book upside down on his own shelf, and then had the subsequently confirmed associated thought that the client may have had an emotionally significant loss of a pregnancy (Reik, 1948). Such a therapeutic event can be viewed as the therapist's neural networks being influenced by the client in ways of which the therapist is unaware, ways that have great therapeutic relevance. The therapist in Reik's example accessed this influence by attending to implicit activities between neural networks in his own brain.

The therapist's awareness of a connection being made does not demand that it be stated or believed; only that it be considered as potentially related to the client's process and possibly useful in the course of treatment. This is congruent with the recommendation made in the chapter on emotion that the client be helped to view emotions and intuitions as information rather than requirements for action. The therapist's conscious decision-making regarding interventions to use remains the guide to determining what ideas to accept as potentially credible and what ideas not to accept. Conscious decision-making also guides the choice regarding whether to express the new awareness to the client.

The statement by the therapist, "Something just popped into my head", has been found in clinical interactions to be a useful introduction to sharing with the client the ideas or images that have occurred to the therapist. The therapist can explain to the client that, similarly to the way the client has been encouraged to observe what pops into the client's own head, the therapist can experience potentially useful ideas as popping into the therapist's head and then share those ideas with the client.

Some of the ideas available to be shared may clearly appear to the therapist to have low potential for unexpected negative responses on the part of the client; other ideas may be assessed by the therapist as having potential to hurt or overwhelm the client. If the client has consistently demonstrated the capacity to cope with strong emotions, then the therapist can predict that if she reports that feeling really sad just popped into her head, the client will be able to cope effectively with such a provocative statement. However, if the client has shown unexpected lability at times, the therapist can choose not to share the idea that has popped into the therapist's head, instead waiting for a more appropriate time or selecting a more appropriate manner for presentation. For example, intellectualized description of an insight may be less overwhelming than directly identifying the emotions of which the therapist has just become aware.

Ideas that pop into the therapist's awareness will vary with regard to how certain the therapist is that the idea is relevant to what the client is experiencing. If the therapist feels sure the idea is related to the client's functioning, it will be more appropriate to present it. If the therapist is less sure of the relevance of the idea to the client's issues, determinants such as the client's flexibility, emotional resilience, or suggestibility may influence the therapist's decision to share the idea.

The therapist's use of ideas that pop into her head and the discussion of such use can contribute to therapy independently of the content of the ideas themselves. By being willing to respect her own ideas popping into awareness, the therapist is modeling acceptance of being in somewhat less control of internal experiences. This can help the client develop such calm acceptance as well. Sharing what has popped into the therapist's head allows for greater confrontation of provocative ideas while attenuating the emotional intensity of the interpersonal aspect of the confrontation. If the idea has just popped into the therapist's head, the therapist appears less sure of the idea, and the client can experience himself as having more latitude to agree or disagree; accepting or rejecting the idea is equated less with the more emotional process of accepting or rejecting the therapist. One source of defensiveness is thereby avoided even though the idea has been introduced into the therapy process. The client can thoughtfully consider ideas of greater intensity because the client does not feel as controlled by the therapist's presentation. Finally, exploring together what pops into the therapist's head offers a model of how to treat ideas and feelings as information rather than as dictates to action, and allows the client to practice such an approach.

Metaphors are one category of thought that can pop into the therapist's or the client's head. Metaphors frequently involve sensory images characterized by substantial levels of emotion. The images often convey multiple meanings at a variety of levels. In light of the neural network concept, it is understood that multiple aspects of the client's presentation in therapy have combined to trigger a complex image that captures much of the client's experience. For example, if the client develops an image of being stranded on a rock in the middle of a torrential current while in view of a sandy beach in a quiet backwater across the river, the image is likely to capture many aspects of the client's present experience of therapy and the issues that are involved. These issues may include isolation, fear of surrounding chaos, concern regarding being overwhelmed, and doubt regarding ability to progress to a better way of functioning. Exploring actions within the context of the metaphor allows procedural processing to continue to unfold within the client, whereas asking the client what the possible meaning could be of being on the rock is an intervention that will take the client out of procedural, sensory-affect connections and into frontal, executive processing. Either intervention may be useful, depending on the capacities and current functioning of the client.

It is possible that at the same time the client describes a metaphor, the therapist finds a different metaphor or a metaphor with different details coming to mind. In the present example, the therapist may have an image of a rope tied between the isolated rock and the peaceful shore. This would suggest the possibility that the therapist's unconscious awareness of the client includes recognition that the client is open to receiving help even though the client feels isolated and overwhelmed at the moment. The therapist can choose whether to explore this new aspect of functioning at all, to introduce the rope image without intellectual explanation, or introduce the rope with intellectual explanation. Thus, through either the client's or the therapist's metaphoric images various aspects of neural networks related to therapy issues can be explored directly or indirectly. The neural network concept offers a conceptual structure that guides understanding of the relevance of the metaphor, and also guides optimal use of the metaphor.

The use of the therapist's neural networks during the course of therapy brings to consideration the importance of the therapist understanding his or her own issues and thereby being able to monitor the impact of such issues on therapy. Psychoanalytic therapists have advocated this for many years, and have expressed this understanding in the recommendation that the psychoanalytic therapist undergo psychoanalytic therapy as part of training (Paolino, 1981). "Therapist, know thyself!" When an image or thought pops into the head of the therapist, it is an expression of neural processes within the therapist. These processes reflect a mixture of current input from the client and past experiences of the therapist. For example, if the therapist is aware that issues of loneliness are important concerns in the therapist's own life, he should be less inclined to interpret ideas related to loneliness as emanating from presentations of the client. If the therapist is clear that his own issues of loneliness do not seem similar to the images of loneliness popping into his head while working with the client, it is more likely that the issues are emerging as a result of information derived from the client.

The therapist's brain functioning influences therapy with the client. Awareness of brain processes within the therapist improves the therapist's ability to use his or her own brain during therapy, and offers novel ways to improve clients' understanding and acceptance of themselves. Discussions with the client regarding using the therapist's brain processes are one way in which focus on the brain can be directly shared with the client during therapy. The next chapter explores how discussions with the client regarding the client's own brain processes can also contribute to psychotherapy.

18

Communicating with clients through neuroscience

The discussion of applying neuroscience to psychological therapies has thus far emphasized the effects of this approach on the therapist's conceptualizations of the client and on the therapist's decisions regarding interventions. In Chapter 17 on the therapist's neuroscience it was briefly discussed how descriptions to the client of the therapist's own brain processes may facilitate communication with the client regarding events in psychotherapy. In fact, clinical experience suggests that one of the most powerful effects of adopting a neuroscience view of psychotherapy is that this view offers an effective basis for communicating with the client and helping the client participate actively in the therapy process.

The application of brain-based models, interventions, and explanations during discussions with clients can change clients' experiences of therapy in a number of ways (see Table 18.1). Discussing brain function can increase clients' understanding of their own psychological strengths and weaknesses, can improve clients' understanding of the therapy process, and can reduce anxiety associated with problems and interventions. Clinical experience has suggested that when clients focus on brain functions rather than personal problems they tend to maintain more positive views of themselves and participate in the therapy process more effectively. Discussing brain

Table 18.1. Effects of integrating neuroscience into discussions with clients

- Improves clients' understanding of themselves
- Offers concrete explanations
- Heightens familiarity and orientation
- Improves clients' understanding of therapy process
- Provides rationales for interventions
- Limits extent of the problem
- Separates client identity from problem
- Empowers client

processes also appears to facilitate an integrated perception of various aspects of intervention, thereby improving clients' abilities to cooperate with multiple mental health care providers during the course of treatment. Consideration of the various effects of communicating with clients regarding brain function can help therapists take the greatest advantage of these effects while also helping therapists maintain acute awareness of how brain-based interventions may complement traditional treatment programs.

Describing patterns of brain functioning that may account for clients' experiences can help clients understand their problems more clearly. They can begin to understand how certain external influences trigger specific areas of the brain that are associated with specific types of internal experience, and they can more easily understand how subsequent behaviors and reactions then unfold. If a client complains of repeated experiences of irrational panic whenever a relationship becomes strong, and if it has been established the client has a history of repeated experiences of abandonment beginning at an early age, then it can be explained to the client that implicit connections have likely been established between neural networks associated with establishing relationships and neural networks associated with loss accompanied by panic. As a result, whenever close personal relationships begin to develop, panic is triggered and it disrupts current relationships even though the panic may not be valid in the current setting. If a different client has overwhelming emotional reactions to a variety of stressful environmental events, and if it has been identified that emotional lability has been observed in family members in previous generations, it can be explained that any emotional trigger may set off a genetically derived, poorly modulated affect system that then drives extreme behaviors that do not fit the situations in which the client currently functions. The first of these examples involves developmental history while the second refers to genetic endowment. In either case, explaining related brain processes can provide the client and the therapist with a shared understanding that guides them toward developing positive expectations, goals, and interventions.

Explanations such as the ones just described can help a variety of clients who have different intellectual capacities and educational backgrounds understand in a relatively unbroken flow the connections between environmental triggers, internal experiences, and subsequent behaviors. Clients' experiences in the world begin to make sense to them in ways that use their own levels of insight to integrate multiple aspects of their own functioning.

These explanations are concrete, and therefore can be described in simple, easily visualized steps. For example, the therapist could offer the fairly simple explanation that when the client meets a man who has characteristics of his father who physically beat the client when the client was younger, the similarities between current and past visual images trigger connections with feelings of pain and fear that have been repeatedly rehearsed in the past. The brain-based explanation offers a rationale for the fact that even though the client is now a tall, muscular male, the client experiences "unreasonable" anxiety in the presence of men similar to his father.

Furthermore, a complex pattern of brain activity associated with experiences and behavior can be offered at a level of detail that meets the needs and taps the capabilities of more sophisticated clients. An anxiety neurosis could be explained to be the result of repeated rejection by both parents incurred because the client was not gratifying to the two narcissistic, intellectual parents. Neural networks composed of images of valued others could be conceptualized as triggering anxiety because the brain's warning system recognizes that the person is approaching a situation (emotional bonding with valued others) that has led to the pain of rejection in the past. It could then be explained that the client has subsequently learned to manage the anxiety by working hard in the client's career as an academician. Engaging in academic work creates connections with the original images of intellectual parents while also helping the client escape relationships by retreating into academic research. In the course of therapy with a psychologically sophisticated client the client would be encouraged to notice what pops into the client's head during therapy sessions as well as between sessions, thereby allowing further perceptions and memories subtly connected to the pattern of rejection to emerge into consciousness, that is, into hippocampal/frontal processing centers, where such memories and perceptions can lead to change over time.

When working with various people associated with the same clinical case, concrete, brain-based conceptualizations in the mind of the therapist can provide the basis for simplistic or complex presentations of the same problem, depending on the capacities of the various people who receive the explanation of the problem. In working with a child who has trouble with behavior in the classroom, it can be explained to the child that when a test is handed out it pushes the brain's fear button, and then the child reacts by doing things to disrupt the class. It can be explained to the parents that a genetically-based difficulty processing visual, verbal information has led to the development of an expectation of failure through repeated rehearsal so that now the child panics in the presence of only moderately challenging written work; the child's subsequent behavioral disruptions then help reduce the child's panic by changing from neural networks associated with panic to networks associated with aggression in the classroom. Moving from one level to another of brain-based description of a client's problem helps ensure that the different levels of conceptualization integrate well with each other. Vague constructs such as superego or introjected self-object contain much subtle information in the mind of the therapist that does not appear to be easily translated into varying levels of understanding for different clients. This seems particularly true when clients are limited with regard to abstract reasoning.

Furthermore, abstract conceptualizations tend to incorporate different subtleties for different professionals or clients in ways that add significantly to problems in clarity of communication. It seems possible that there may not be helpful, concrete, brain-based descriptions that capture the essence of the most sophisticated understanding of a client's intrapsychic functioning. However, it seems likely that the risk of losing understanding through use of highly abstract concepts during communication with clients will be greater than the likelihood of gaining understanding, when compared with brain-based modeling.

Concrete explanations appear to be less threatening than many of the vague terms used in dynamic and interpersonal psychotherapies. A neural network can be described as simply a set of neurons throughout the brain that have fired simultaneously repeatedly over time. People may or may not be aware of the network, depending on how active it has been recently, how much of the network is stimulated by current events, or how consistently anxiety disrupts the activation of the given network. Such a description is less vague and less threatening than being told that repressed memories are activating punitive superego mechanisms that lead to masochistic inclinations.

At the present time it appears that combining brain-based explanations with explanations founded on more traditional schools of therapy can offer the potential for in-depth understanding in complicated cases. The repressed memories just referenced might be described as neural networks that include a pattern of triggering anxiety followed by self-deprecatory actions that relieve the anxiety. Exploration of the associations generated in connection with the experience of hurting oneself might bring to light a sense of being connected with loved but punitive parents, thereby providing a more concrete neural hypothesis based on conceptualizations originally founded on traditional theory. Such an integration of brain concepts with traditional theory can reduce the mysteriousness that seems unnecessary while maintaining a level of sophistication of understanding that can improve the likelihood of change.

Brain-based explanations of psychological problems and the therapy process increase clients' awareness of "where they are" in the flow of perceiving external information, processing experiences based on current and previous learning, and behaving in accordance with connections within various neural networks. Such awareness can provide a sense of familiarity that is soothing even when problems have not been resolved. As previously described, novelty, that is, lack of familiarity, can independently trigger anxiety that can disrupt adaptive functioning within the brain by stimulating generalized arousal; this arousal can interfere with the activation of discrete neural networks associated with positive coping. If lack of familiarity can be countered by brain-based conceptualizations, clients will move more successfully toward improvement even when there are problems along the way.

For example, if a client recognizes that social anxiety is likely to disrupt thinking and result in the client saying inappropriate things in a social setting, the client can be encouraged to acknowledge that such behaviors are likely even though the client is aware that the eventual goal is to change such behaviors. It can be explained that network connections established during earlier procedural learning continue to include connections between affect and undesired motor responding; as a result, disruptive motor behaviors such as inappropriate comments can be triggered by old procedural memory patterns that still emerge even though the client's plans, which reflect new networks in the declarative, frontal/hippocampal system, focus on producing more appropriate behaviors. The client will not be surprised by the client's own failures, and will be able to maintain a proactive attitude and approach toward behavioral change despite procedural memories still influencing behavior in a negative way.

Brain-based discussions with clients appear to go beyond just reducing anxiety by increasing clients' familiarity with their own intrapsychic processes and with general characteristics of treatment. Discussions of the neuroscience of treatment rationales appear to increase clients' understanding of the specific processes involved in treatment, thereby improving compliance and quality of effort. Increased understanding of the processes involved makes it more likely that clients will be willing to engage in activities that are often accompanied by anxiety but are also likely to contribute to change over time. For example, exposure strategies in behavior therapy offer rationales for the client confronting feared stimuli: a client can be told that research has found exposure treatment to lead to improvement. However, such rationales do not include a clear explanation of the internal experiences of which the client is likely to become aware in the course of exposure treatment. A brain-based explanation might describe the habituation process at the level of intercellular connections, so that the client would better understand how prolonged exposure to an extremely uncomfortable situation is likely to lead to reduced numbers of connections between the cue and the response, thus leading to behavioral and emotional improvement. A brain-based rationale could also include a description of the process of repeatedly connecting frontal brain control mechanisms to old neural networks, thereby pairing positive decision-making procedures with a previously automatic anxiety response. This combination of explanations can make it clear to the client why activation of both new and old neural patterns is necessary in order for change to occur. The client can thus understand better why complete and persistent exposure is required in order for change to occur. It has been observed during clinical work that improved participation in treatment is a result of such understanding.

Describing complex psychological problems in terms of the various brain systems involved supports individual rationales for each of several interventions used during psychotherapy. A rationale for each intervention can be provided in light of the brain system being targeted. Working with a client diagnosed with Borderline Personality Disorder offers an example of such an approach. When working with such a client, relaxation training can be described as reducing overall levels of arousal that can trigger emotionality and disrupt functioning. Rationales for medications can be given in light of the specific problem systems identified: Selective Serotonin Reuptake Inhibitor (SSRI) antidepressant medications can be identified as improving mood, while the use of valproate and other mood stabilizers' can be described as reducing emotional reactivity (Scahill & Martin, 2001), leaving the person more able to use frontal executive functions effectively. Triggers for maladaptive dissociative coping can be identified so that the client feels less pathological when such coping unfolds despite the client's best efforts to stop related behaviors and thinking. The tendency for emotions to overwhelm logical thinking can be accounted for in a description of the interactions between new, hippocampally-based function and old histories of maladaptive emotionally intense procedural learning; such a description can provide a rationale for hope despite the long learning curve required in order to change such patterns enough to yield successful behaviors. Clinical observations have indicated that increased specificity of rationales results in increased ability on the borderline client's part to recognize where the client is in the process of psychotherapy and to understand why a specific aspect of treatment should be undertaken even though the intense emotions experienced by the client scream to avoid or undermine the intervention. Specific reference to the slow nature of implicit learning and unlearning can support acceptance of the slow nature of change. References to brain systems can also help the borderline client accept and cope more effectively with emotions that do not match the conscious, frontal insights and goals the client adopts. Brain-based descriptions can thus help attenuate the extreme responses that are typical during work with clients diagnosed with Borderline Personality Disorder.

Beyond affecting clients' views of problems and interventions, explanations of the neural basis of problems appears to alter clients' views of themselves. Explicit identification of brain systems likely to underlie specific patterns of psychological dysfunction helps reduce the extent to which clients view their problems as defects in the whole person. "I have Bipolar Disorder" is a statement implying global inadequacy of a person. When the disorder is presented as a problem with an over-active affect system, clients are more likely to maintain a sense that a part of the self, the frontal/hippocampal system for example, is available to work toward developing better control over affective responses. Furthermore, the client can be helped to recognize that prosocial thoughts and behaviors involve other areas of the brain and are real and sincerely held parts of the self even though emotions frequently result in behaviors that seem opposed to these positive qualities. Feelings of love for family and friends, wishes to help others, and wishes to achieve positive goals can all be accepted and believed more readily by clients when the mood disorder is conceived as a breakdown in a specific brain system. Elements of positive self-esteem within clients are more likely to be forthcoming, and such positive elements in life can provide support to clients working toward positive change.

Brain-based explanations emphasizing that psychological problems are the result of dysfunction in discrete, limited areas of the brain also help people associated with clients to perceive problems as limited rather than global. Parents, teachers, spouses, and others working with clients have been observed to shift from perceiving a client as a mean or bad person to identifying specific areas of difficulty accompanied by multiple aspects of positive functioning. When parents and teachers are helped to understand bipolar disorder as the result of dysfunction in affect systems they can then begin to accept their bipolar child's statements of caring and wishing to do better as honest and sincere rather than manipulative. When the husband of an abused female client recognizes that implicit neural connections between affect and sexual touching are not readily controlled by the client, and that change will occur slowly over time after multiple rehearsals of substitute experiences, the husband can become more hopeful and more helpful with regard to treatment. In the same way that understanding the neural substrates of psychological difficulties helps clients acknowledge positive qualities in themselves, so, too, can neural explanations allow those around clients to do the same thing.

When psychological problems are viewed as related to problems in specific brain systems rather than results of global dysfunction, the client's sense of identity as a person is separated from the problem itself. During the past two decades there has been increasing awareness of the connections between psychopathology and the biochemical nature of brain function. This awareness has been used in attempts to reduce the moral shame associated with psychological or psychiatric disorders; the term "chemical imbalance" has been offered to clients in a basic attempt to demystify and destigmatize psychiatric disorders. However, chemical imbalance has been observed to be interpreted by clients as an imbalance throughout the brain, so even though the aspect of moral degeneration has been reduced, the perception of global dysfunction has remained. Identification of the specific areas of the brain related to the client's difficulties reduces the globalization of the problem, allowing more opportunity for the development of a positive sense of identity despite the presence of areas of poor function. For example, describing the systems and behaviors associated with attention problems is less pejorative than being told, "You have Attention Deficit/ Hyperactivity Disorder". Similarly, describing a client's Bipolar II Disorder as a problem with the emotion switch being all or none rather than operating as a rheostat is less threatening than telling the client, "Your Bipolar II Disorder is a result of a chemical imbalance".

Focusing on specific brain systems during therapy empowers clients by giving them specific positive goals and directions while simultaneously emphasizing that only specific, limited parts of the brain are the focus of change rather than the whole self. The emphasis on positive client qualities derives from the fact that any given intervention relies on parts of the brain that are operating effectively in support of positive change. The therapeutic goal of changing brain function thus automatically, in both implicit and explicit ways, focuses on client strengths and assets throughout change. Frontal, rational executive systems can be described as supporting insight that can facilitate change even though the client still experiences herself as being driven by emotions and by previously developed implicit memories associated with maladaptive patterns. Applying relaxation skills to threatening situations connects neural centers related to calmness with sensory systems that have previously been associated with emotional pain or fear. The sense of unfamiliarity or being lost that often accompanies behaving in ways that are at odds with conscious awareness and intent can be reduced by understanding the relationships between declarative and nondeclarative memory systems. As a result, the influence of a major source of negative affect is reduced and, at the same time, the influence of brain systems underlying positive self-management are emphasized. Conscious, declarative neural networks characterized by taking action, persisting, and maintaining direction are facilitated because of the directive to focus on activating positive systems rather than to be solely invested in turning off negative experiences.

Focus on brain systems offers a framework within which to discuss with clients the integration of medical interventions into the change process. Often clients express the belief that they are weaker because they have to rely on medications for help with change. When medications can be identified as helping manage a specific brain system rather than the brain as a whole, the extent to which taking such medications undermines a person's positive view of himself is reduced. When problems are identified as being the result of malfunctioning in a certain system, then change associated with medication can be described in terms of how medication affects the specific system involved. This offers understanding on the part of the client, and therefore greater likelihood of knowledgeable acceptance of medication interventions.

Identifying brain mechanisms affected by medications may also suggest more effective ways of taking advantage of improvements facilitated by medication. Anti-anxiety medications can be described as reducing generalized activity in the brain, thereby allowing the person to think more clearly since brain systems are no longer so disrupted by anxiety. It can be explained that when brain functioning is less disrupted by anxiety it becomes possible to concentrate on specific problem-solving strategies more effectively. Clients can be helped to see that it may also be important not to medicate away all distressing aspects of a situation since confronting the distressing feeling state gives the client opportunities to pair new adaptive responses with previous negative feelings. If medication reduces all anxiety in a situation, it would be hypothesized that the person would never have the opportunity to habituate to the maladaptive negative pattern.

In a different example, the use of stimulant medications to activate attention systems can be explained as allowing the person to take advantage of the valuable neural connections that have previously been available but untapped. This can be phrased as, "The medication does not make you smarter; it just gives you the chance to use more effectively the neural connections that are already available". This concept can be used to help clients who are taking medications continue to take both credit and responsibility for their own decisions and behaviors. It can be pointed out that the medication does not turn people into nicer people; rather, if the person wants to do the right thing, the medication allows the person to do it more easily and more consistently.

Researchers have presented PET scan results showing how stimulant medications support the whole brain running smoothly rather than having only portions of the brain running when medication is not present (Amen, 2004). The image of more of the brain being turned on as a result of use of stimulants can be offered to the client as indicating that using stimulant medications probably allows more of the brain, and more of the person, to be available instead of triggering the brain and the person to become something the person previously was not before the use of medication.

Descriptions of how the brain works can also help people understand how using medications may help the brain develop new and better connections that will remain even when medication is discontinued. Often clients wonder if using stimulant medications will mean the person will not be able to use what is learned while medicated unless medication is present in the future. It can be pointed out that attention systems help to prime or activate specific patterns of neural firing associated with goal-directed learning. As a result, stronger connections can be established throughout the brain when attention is maintained with stimulant medications. It is hypothesized that when stimulant medication is absent at a later date, the stronger connections developed between various neurons in the neural network as a result of previous higher levels of attention will still leave the connections more likely to fire in the future even in the absence of stimulant medications. For example, if a student has attention problems that interfere with the development of reading skills, it can be pointed out that if the student learns to read while taking stimulant medications, the underlying neural wiring supporting the skills learned will remain even when medication is discontinued.

The use of medications to help manage anxiety can similarly be described in light of the neural systems involved. If a person is so anxious that whenever thoughts about a particular topic occur, the anxiety disrupts focus or triggers avoidance, the person cannot change the pattern of responding because new experiences and thoughts cannot be paired with the old pattern when it is deactivated through habituation. An appropriate level of anti-anxiety medication can allow the person to maintain engagement with the anxiety provoking neural patterns and thereby work on changing them. In this way the use of anti-anxiety medications can be understood by the client to encourage competence and active coping while not establishing a requirement that the medication be present in order to activate all aspects of improvement obtained during the period medication was being used.

Conceptualizations based on brain function offer new ways to communicate with clients during therapy. The concrete nature of connections between brain function and clients' experiences and behaviors helps clients develop better understanding of psychological problems, psychological strengths, and processes that unfold during therapy. This understanding can be the basis for increased cooperation, reduced resistance, and more effective client participation in the process of psychotherapy. A brain-based approach can facilitate clients becoming more active and intentional in their participation in therapy. Brain-based understanding can also help clients analyze experiences outside the therapist's office and apply understanding of brain functioning during the development of more adaptive day-to-day responses. As therapy unfolds, helping clients approach problems by considering brain functions involved can offer a framework within which clients are better able to collaborate with the therapist while the client and the therapist work to achieve change in life.

19

Integrating traditional therapies

Beyond offering a free-standing framework for conducting therapy, brain functions and systems can provide a framework within which traditional therapies can be understood and integrated. Since all change in psychotherapy is hypothesized to be based on changes in the way the brain takes in, processes, and responds to information from the world around the individual, it makes sense that traditional models of psychotherapy can be considered in light of brain systems involved (Kandel, 1998). Knowledge of brain systems can help elucidate processes of therapy within each traditional model while also making clear how different models relate to each other. The result can be an integration of the strengths of the various traditional models. This integration can facilitate shifting from one treatment model to another in a seamless way, thereby supporting more effective overall intervention. At the same time, communication between therapists operating within the confines of different traditional models can be facilitated, offering another way in which treatment can be enhanced.

Psychodynamic, behavioral, cognitive–behavioral, and Gestalt theories will be considered as examples during the present discussion. In addition, pharmacotherapy will also be discussed as a form of intervention. For current purposes, only selected elements of each school of intervention will be examined, since more complete analysis of connections between brain systems and the respective schools would be far more complex than the present venue permits.

Each psychotherapy theory can be considered within the neuroscience framework developed in previous chapters. In the present chapter the framework will be used to guide examination of the elements of brain function that are actively engaged during traditional interventions. These elements include implicit and explicit memory processes, developmental contributions, and the details encapsulated in Figures 1.1 and 9.1. In addition, it will also be clearly identified what aspects of the brain model tend not to be addressed or intentionally activated by individual traditional models and interventions. The final result can be a roadmap of connections between psychotherapy and the brain, and this roadmap can help identify pathways of intervention followed by each school of therapy while pinpointing intersections and locating divergences between theories.

One aspect of brain functioning highlighted in the current neuroscience model is usually given little consideration by any of the traditional theories. Patterns of strength and weakness in cognitive processing that are typically assessed using intellectual, achievement, and neuropsychological testing are usually not addressed during assessment and intervention guided by traditional theories of psychotherapy. Problems with attention, relative strengths in verbal and nonverbal arenas, and presence or absence of difficulty at various levels of integration of verbal and nonverbal information are commonly assessed in a minimal way through observation of thought flow, judgment, or insight. Verbal and nonverbal avenues of motor expression are most often assessed as evidence of arousal, anxiety, emotion, or patterns related to history and underlying psychological issues. Furthermore, during therapy, observations of motivation, decision-making, and other frontal, executive processes may be interpreted as evidence of underlying emotional or psychodynamic contributors to clients' chosen behaviors when, instead, the processes observed actually reflect characteristics of the client's cognitive capacities.

Strengths and weaknesses in various channels of cognitive processing can greatly influence the extent to which change can be facilitated using these channels. A person who is much stronger nonverbally than verbally is likely to process experiences in areas of the brain that have few connections with words and verbal meaning. Despite inability to verbalize understanding, such a person may nevertheless understand experiences in ways that are insightful and complex. Within the context of psychodynamic therapy the failure to generate verbal expression of underlying issues may be interpreted as defensive even though the real reason for lack of production is lack of ability in channels of cognitive functioning that are necessary to support such expression. Within the framework of cognitive behavioral therapy, development of new patterns of verbal self-talk may have little impact on a client's functioning because verbalization has little connection to the nonverbal imagery that typically triggers behaviors in a person weak in verbal processing. Failure to consider the effects of cognitive strengths and weaknesses on processing during therapy may result in misinterpretations followed by disruptions in the flow of therapy.

Psychodynamic theories

Psychodynamic psychotherapy is a complex, relatively well-defined approach to psychotherapy, and it contains several specific constructs that can be usefully analyzed in light of a neuroscience framework. These constructs include free association, transference, and the combination of anxiety, defense, and the unconscious. Connections between brain processes and the psychodynamic model as a whole will be discussed, and then individual elements will be examined with regard to brain processes involved.

Psychodynamic intervention is a stepwise process (see Gabbard, 2004). The first step is to activate the various neural network patterns supporting maladaptive thoughts, emotions, and behaviors. Often these patterns include procedural connections that have been repeatedly rehearsed but that have few connections to declarative, conscious processes. Once these networks supporting maladaptive processes are activated, ties are established between past patterns and current function; if current incoming stimuli do not match the old maladaptive patterns, the connections in the old pattern begin to weaken. Networks including conscious, declarative processes are activated simultaneously with the old maladaptive networks. The client is then helped to recognize the maladaptive nature of previously developed patterns; networks underlying conscious understanding become connected to previously unconscious neural patterns, thereby shifting the way the previously unconscious patterns influence functioning. Finally, the process of psychodynamic intervention allows the client to intentionally activate new, more adaptive neural patterns in response to experiencing and recognizing the maladaptive aspects of previous patterns.

A primary task in psychodynamic psychotherapy is to elucidate patterns of brain connection established over the course of development and experience. Free association is the main strategy used in this elucidation (Fenichel, 1945). Noticing what pops into your head is a way of describing this strategy. The goal of this strategy is to reduce activation of frontal, executive, analytic processes that can disrupt the unfolding of implicit, unconscious connections between one network and the next. As a result of allowing these implicit connections to become active enough to reach the level of conscious awareness, they become available for subsequent frontal executive analysis and influence. Because free association fosters activation of procedural, implicit memory connections, and because free association allows the full neural network to unfold, psychodynamic therapies are likely to activate many of the client's old, maladaptive neural networks. Lower brain systems affecting arousal, mood systems, anxiety systems, attachment centers, verbal and nonverbal connections, frontal/executive connections, and motor systems are all likely to be activated during free association (see Figures 1.1 and 9.1). Psychodynamic conceptualizations offer elegant delineations of the variety of maladaptive patterns that can occur (Fenichel, 1945; Gabbard, 2004). Connections between sensory experiences and emotions can be discovered, and ways in which past patterns prime current experiences can be identified. It appears that the primary avenue of change within psychodynamic theories is the simultaneous activation of old negative patterns in the presence of competing adaptive experiences and conscious, declarative insights that subsequently become connected to the old neural networks, leading to change in the experience of the old patterns (Gabbard, 2004).

These therapeutic processes are often explored and resolved as aspects of the relationship between the therapist and the client in the course of psychodynamic psychotherapy (Gabbard, 2004). Neural networks related to previous experiences prime the client to develop a similar set of perceptions of the therapist. This set of perceptions is identified as "the transference", and the identification and resolution of historically maladaptive patterns often occurs during the development and "working through" of the transference. Bringing such patterns into conscious awareness in the context of the relationship with the therapist is conceived within the present model to integrate frontal/hippocampal systems of conscious, declarative memory into previously established implicit and explicit patterns, thereby shifting the ways the old, maladaptive patterns unfold in the future. Change occurs through developing awareness of underlying patterns and through having competing experiences. Insight (Fenichel, 1945) as well as "corrective emotional experiences" (Alexander & French, 1946) in the relationship with the therapist contribute to change in the client's functioning.

Brain-based conceptualizations offer an understanding of the nature of anxiety, defenses, repression, and "the unconscious" that is more flexible than the understanding offered by traditional psychodynamic theories. Psychodynamic theories of anxiety suggest that experiences in the past that have led to fear or pain begin to serve as triggers or "signals" for anxiety, and that the person develops ways of behaving or thinking that avoid or reduce the anxiety (Fenichel, 1945). The original pattern tying external experience to emotional pain becomes unconscious because the defensive patterns unfold before the original pattern is complete; the defensive pattern blocks out awareness of the original painful experience. Despite being unconscious, the pattern still influences day-to-day behavior. It is implied in this psychodynamic approach that the pattern to be avoided was originally conscious.

The neuroscience brain model suggests that unconscious, maladaptive patterns may or may not have gone through a process of repression. Procedural connections between sensory input and affect may have been established without hippocampal activity, either because that specific pattern of connection was never a focus of awareness, because it occurred during the first several years of life before long-term memory processes were active, or because the intensity of the negative pattern was so high that hippocampal, conscious recording of the event never occurred (LeDoux, 1996). Such a non-repressed procedural memory would be expected to influence brain activity even though the person has never been consciously aware of the original pattern or the experience that led to it. The pattern is unconscious without ever being repressed. Exploration of such a maladaptive pattern would be considered to be discovering rather than recovering.

Furthermore, the novelty monitor proposed by Gray (1982) suggests the presence of triggers for anxiety that are quite separate from the repression process. As the person moves toward new functioning the experience is likely to be identified as novel by the internal monitoring system, and anxiety can be the result. Such anxiety can be misinterpreted by therapists or clients as meaning that underlying maladaptive patterns remain to be explored. An inappropriate search for sources can follow. However, it is possible that such anxiety is the expectable response of a person beginning to behave using brain patterns that are adaptive but unfamiliar. Adding such a consideration to traditional psychodynamic understanding of anxiety offers greater understanding and flexibility.

Conceptualizing events during psychodynamic psychotherapy in terms of brain systems involved may shift the nature of the therapy process to some degree. The uncovering of old negative patterns during traditional analytic psychotherapy is accompanied by abstract rather than concrete explanations of how such patterns are likely to operate within the person, so the likelihood of the client feeling overwhelmed by the experiences seems high. If the therapy process is experienced as vague or mysterious the client is likely to feel out of control, vulnerable, and dependent. This is especially true when strong emotions and high levels of anxiety are parts of the networks being activated. Traditionally, psychodynamic theories have conceived of the working through of such feelings as being a keystone of the treatment. However, the intensity of such feelings in treatment may be a non-critical secondary result of lacking a more understandable explanatory model of the way the client is functioning. Conceptualizing the various client patterns in terms of the brain systems involved may reduce the tendency for such feelings to develop. Reference to brain function has been found to facilitate moving back and forth between free association and frontal, executive self-direction (ego control) in ways that allow exploration and adaptation to take place in flexible, effective ways. Clinical observations have indicated that transference is still likely to develop in the course of therapy, but the brain-based model allows for the therapist and client to collaborate in the modulation of associated reactions so that the client is not overwhelmed. This allows the client to gain a sense of self-efficacy and security while also being aware of the issues being addressed.

The reduction in being overwhelmed may facilitate more rapid development of "ego" controls. That is, concrete, brain-based explanations may facilitate more rapid development of frontal, executive, declarative processing of situations, accompanied by pairing of this processing with old, maladaptive patterns. The process of moving between exploration and management of brain systems associated with maladaptive functioning is a process that emphasizes self-efficacy. Self-efficacy thus begins to be paired with the experience of the maladaptive pattern. The choice can be made for the client to remain engaged in the maladaptive pattern for longer or shorter periods of time, with the longer immersion being used when exploration is the primary goal and when the client has the psychological ability to bear such immersion.

In addition to the self-efficacy and skill building fostered by moving back and forth between uncovering and managing, consideration of brain systems promotes the active development of competing patterns that can replace or modify old patterns. If a client uncovers a pattern of becoming overly dependent in relationships throughout life, the client can be encouraged to imagine novel ways of behaving in those settings, and then to allow the old patterns and newly imagined patterns to exist in awareness at the same time. This is hypothesized to facilitate hippocampal long-term potentiation processes (Kandel, 2000) that can support insight and rapid change (O'Keefe & Nadel, 1978). The client can be encouraged to imagine taking steps to independently take care of needs rather than waiting for others to take care of those needs. Simply considering the idea of such change while also considering the old need for dependence is expected to lead to change in the experience of the old patterns, even before the client begins to take independent action. Brain-based conceptualizations thus offer a context that supports facilitation of positive development in more active ways than would be prescribed in accordance with traditional psychodynamic theories.

Analysis of psychodynamic therapy in terms of brain processes involved highlights the extent to which psychodynamic interventions typically do not include the active development of new neural networks to replace old, maladaptive networks. Traditional psychodynamic interventions do not readily prescribe substitute beliefs, concepts, or behaviors that can replace the maladaptive patterns explored, relying instead on the client to independently develop replacement patterns. Viewed within the current neuroscience model, the lack of focus on developing substitute adaptive networks adds unnecessarily to anxiety in the client while also interfering with the completion of change.

It is useful to summarize psychodynamic therapy in terms of the elements of the Big Picture model (Figure 9.1). Psychodynamic therapies do not typically focus on cognitive elements including attention, verbal and non-verbal processing systems, or levels of integration available to the client within each system. Psychodynamic therapy emphasizes patterns, that is, neural networks, that developed in the past and currently influence clients' behaviors within and outside the therapy session. These networks or patterns include arousal, emotions, anxiety, attitudes, goals, and motor activity including speech and behavior. Change primarily occurs through developing declarative, explicit awareness and new patterns of emotional reaction, and then combining these new patterns with old patterns, thereby encouraging change in old patterns. Psychodynamic interventions do not emphasize clear and concrete guidance in the development of new patterns of thought and behavior, relying instead on the client to produce such patterns independently as part of the process of working through the old patterns.

Behavioral theories

Behavior therapy and modification includes interventions and conceptualizations that range from "radical behaviorist" applied behavior analysis to social learning theory that identifies the importance of cognitive mediational activities (Krasner, 1990). The term radical behaviorist refers to an exclusive focus on the environmental influences on a person's behavior, eschewing consideration of a person's internal processes as a focus during the process of behavior change. Such a view is substantially different from views held by cognitive-behavioral therapists who emphasize cognitive mediational processes in their understanding of change (Dobson, 2003). The differences between these conceptualizations are particularly striking since both approaches are included under the umbrella of "behavior therapy/modification" (Krasner, 1990). For the purpose of examining connections between brain function and types of therapy intervention, behavior therapies and cognitive-behavioral therapies are considered separately. Classical conditioning strategies and operant behavior modification paradigms are considered as examples of behavior therapies, while cognitive restructuring and constructivist theories are considered under the heading cognitive-behavioral therapies.

Classical conditioning models have been used in the development of effective interventions for reducing anxiety and associated avoidance that occur in response to specific sensory input. The use of "reciprocal inhibition" to treat simple phobias offers a primary example of such intervention (Wolpe, 1958). Reciprocal inhibition involves presenting the client with an environmental event that triggers high levels of anxiety, and subsequently training the client to achieve a relaxed state that is then associated with the external stimuli that previously triggered anxiety.

Reciprocal inhibition can be examined in light of brain systems likely to be involved. An external stimulus activates sensory systems that subsequently activate anxiety responses by way of Gray's (1982) septal-hippocampal monitoring system; neural networks underlying an anxiety response are then stimulated to fire. A competing relaxation response is then activated and paired with the incoming stimuli that initially triggered the anxiety. At the same time, the old pattern of fear response to the stimulus is habituated. The avoidance behavior becomes less frequent and intense, and the new network no longer includes severe anxiety in response to presentation of the original stimuli. Treatment for phobias, for example, the fear of heights, can be very concise and time limited following such an intervention program.

Examination of behavior intervention approaches in light of the currently offered model of brain function in psychotherapy (Figure 1.1) helps identify multiple aspects of brain function not addressed by behavioral analysis. Complex internal network patterns are not considered relevant, with focus being maintained instead on the connections within the sensory stimulus–fear–avoidance pattern. The values of insight, declarative memory processes, unidentified procedural memory connections, attachment processes, and developmental issues tend to be minimized or ignored completely. The assumption underlying the approach is that if the behavior is changed, the related internal processes will also change without being addressed directly. Complicated internal triggering patterns are likely not to be effectively identified and as a result the interventions may fail to address important aspects of stimulus events (Lang, 1979). Connections between stimuli and emotions other than fear are also not likely to be identified or addressed.

Frontal, declarative processing systems are used during behavioral interventions to identify basic connections between environmental stimuli and fear responses, and subsequently to guide the exposure program; however, frontal awareness is not used to shift internal patterns of feeling and thought. Because the focus of the intervention process is on external stimuli rather than on the process of interpreting the fear, it is likely the client and therapist will fail to understand the contributions of attachment or other developmental issues to problems and their resolution. The tendency for behavioral interventions to focus on the current behavioral patterns is likely to result in little consideration being given to the implications of early experiences in the context of brain development. This narrow focus increases the likelihood that the nature of the symptom patterns will be misunderstood or inadequately formulated.

Reciprocal inhibition interventions can also be considered in light of the Big Picture. Frontal executive decision-making processes guide the client's engagement in the therapy process. The first task of treatment is the development of relaxation skills. Executive systems intentionally activate motor control of internal bodily activities that support relaxation, leading to proprioceptive input that can later compete with anxiety responses. Once the relaxation response is well established, attention processes are activated in order to support focus on exposure procedures, but the quality of attention capacities is not typically assessed. Sensory input systems are directly activated by the exposure process, but priming of these systems through frontal executive analysis of the problem appears to be minimal. Exposure activates relevant implicit connections without guidance by frontal, executive processes. During basic in vivo exposure procedures sensory information is integrated at varying levels during the course of analyzing incoming information and sending it to systems triggering the anxiety system, but the quality of integration is seldom consciously, intentionally addressed during treatment. Connections between anxiety systems and motor systems are emphasized. Habituation of neural activity in the connections between sensory input, anxiety systems, and motor output is the basis of one aspect of change during reciprocal inhibition. The pairing of relaxation systems with sensory input that originally triggered anxiety establishes a neural pattern that replaces the anxiety response. Arousal systems are affected as part of anxiety networks. Emotion systems and neural network patterns that may be associated with anxiety reactions are disregarded during reciprocal inhibition.

In vivo exposure procedures during reciprocal inhibition present the client with the actual environmental stimuli that trigger anxiety, and only brain systems that funnel information from sensory systems to fear centers and on to motor responses are considered to be activated. It appears that the same implicit memory systems are activated when imaginal presentation of triggering stimuli is used during reciprocal inhibition procedures, although frontal executive systems are relied upon to activate memory traces in various sensory systems rather than assuming that external stimuli trigger relevant sensory systems. Presentation using imagery appears to emphasize declarative memory systems more than does in vivo exposure. In order to stimulate sensory systems involved in imagery, priming based on conscious, declarative processes is used to initiate images. In addition, imaginal exposure is conceived to rely on brain processes that are active rather than passive (Derryberry & Tucker, 1992), so it may be that imaginal exposure increases the establishment of ties between maladaptive patterns and neural systems related to a sense of self-efficacy. This observation derives from consideration of the brain processes involved rather than from consideration of theories contrasting relative efficacy of imaginal and in vivo exposure.

Applied behavior analysis uses operant reinforcement strategies whereby external rewards and punishers are supplied as consequences to selected patterns of experience and behavior (Krasner, 1990). In the case of a reward paradigm, a discriminative stimulus is attended to, registered in the sensory systems, and then integrated into a meaningful cue at some level of complexity. Frontal, executive systems are subsequently activated in order to initiate motor systems that have previously resulted in consequences that increase behavior. Even when the intervention is driven solely by consideration of connections between the client's behavior and the ensuing environmental consequences, some level of internal analysis and decision-making must occur in the client's brain.

Applied behavior analysis may disregard completely elements related to emotion, anxiety, neural networks beyond the stimulus–behavior–consequence connection, genetic contributions, levels of interpersonal attachment, and broad developmental influences (Figures 1.1 and 9.1). The currently offered model of how brain systems affect psychological therapies assumes that clinically significant activity occurs in the various systems that are not directly acknowledged in the radical applied behavior analysis intervention, and that conscious incorporation of understanding of such activity could lead to more effective intervention strategies and to a broader appreciation of how interventions relate to the client's overall functioning.

Cognitive behavioral theories

Cognitive behavioral therapies (CBT) go beyond the stimulus–response connections of behavior therapy to include mediation of functioning by cognitive processes (Dobson, 2003). It is assumed that cognitive activity affects behavior, and that behavior and/or cognitions can be altered by changes in cognitions. Areas of desired change can include behavior, cognitive activity, or both. Substantial range in breadth and complexity is present within this set of therapies, with the term cognitive behavioral therapies subsuming cognitive restructuring, coping skills therapies, and problem-solving therapies. For the purpose of a basic analysis of connect-ions between CBT and brain function, the focus will be on the basic premise that identifying and altering maladaptive thinking can lead to changes in behavior, thought, and mood. More complex examples of CBT interventions will then be considered in order to delineate the range of brain systems and elements that may be activated by CBT interventions.

Identifying and changing cognitions appear to involve identification of elements of maladaptive patterns within the declarative memory system followed by therapy interventions designed to develop new, adaptive patterns that are also based in declarative memory processing systems. Positive self-statements, new social skills, and new problem-solving strategies are paired with input from situations that had previously triggered maladaptive responding. It is assumed that positive cognitive activities will be rewarded by ensuing intrapsychic cognitive events along with positive, rewarding events in the client's environment. CBT focuses on cognitive mediation of all events, so positive external events are rewarding at least in part due to activity in declarative, cognitive mediational systems. Connections with implicit memory systems are given little attention, so little emphasis is given to identifying complex brain patterns that include sensory experience, emotion, attachment, and complex, whole-brain integrations (Figure 1.1).

With regard to the Big Picture model (Figure 9.1) it appears that elements directly activated during implementation of CBT interventions include frontal/executive systems, attention systems focused on detailed steps of verbal reasoning, verbal processing systems relying on varying levels of integration, and motor systems including behaviors selected with guidance from frontal, decision-making systems. Replacement patterns are intentionally paired only with maladaptive patterns that have conscious, declarative elements, so memories stored in non-hippocampal, non-frontal systems are likely not to be directly addressed. It is assumed that changes in other areas of functioning, including arousal, emotion, anxiety, and maladaptive neural networks or patterns (Figure 9.1) will unfold secondarily to changes in the cognitive, declarative processing systems.

More elaborate cognitive behavioral conceptualizations have developed under the umbrella of CBT. These conceptualizations identify the need to develop complete representations of life experiences, that is, schemata, in order to facilitate change (Dobson, 2003; Lang, 1979). These more complete representations can be understood to activate a large of number of brain systems in intentional ways, although identification of brain systems involved is not typically part of the intervention. Exemplifying such approaches, Guidano and his colleagues (Arciero & Guidano, 2000; Guidano & Liotti, 1983) have offered a framework that emphasizes both explicit and tacit processes, including feelings, imagery, and emotional schemata based heavily on development over the lifespan in the context of relationships.

It appears there are multiple similarities between complex CBT conceptualizations and those propounded by therapists operating within modern psychodynamic contexts, and as a result the extent of differences in brain systems activated by these nominally different approaches is relatively small. It seems likely that complex constructivist, CBT interventions focus more explicitly on developing specific new skills for living than do many psychodynamic interventions, so developing new neural networks supporting replacement behaviors seems likely to be more prominent in these interventions than in psychodynamic interventions. It also appears that frontal/executive systems and declarative memory are likely activated more extensively during the development of these new networks than during psychodynamic change. However, similarities in patterns of activation of brain systems highlight the substantial similarities between psychodynamic and constructivist approaches.

Gestalt theories

A primary focus of Gestalt interventions is the facilitation of experiences that express or demonstrate current maladaptive actions, and through these experiences alternative understanding and adaptive actions develop (Smith, 1976). Conscious, intellectual examination of issues is believed to interfere with development of deeper understanding and change. Gestalt therapies overtly emphasize experiencing memories, ideas, and feelings with as many physiological and sensory components involved as possible (Greenberg, 1980). The intense experience of areas of difficulty is hypothesized to promote more complete understanding of problems as well as better problem resolution.

The Gestalt facilitation of experiences related to issues appears to emphasize implicit memory systems more than explicit, declarative brain processes. Sensory systems and memories embedded in them are more likely to be stimulated during Gestalt experiences than during psychotherapy approaches that focus on intellectual analysis (see Figures 1.1 and 9.1). Attention is directed toward senses and emotions rather than toward frontal, executive analysis during periods of therapy when the client is engaged in an intense experience. The intensification of emotions is a primary goal of the experience (Greenberg, 1980), and as emotions become more intense, basic arousal systems are likely to be simultaneously activated. Gestalt experiential techniques appear designed to disregard anxiety rather than address it directly, although the current model of brain functioning suggests that habituation processes are likely to be active during the intense experience of previously unconscious implicit connections. Ties between sensory and motor elements of memory are intentionally activated during Gestalt experiences. Motor processes are encouraged in the Gestalt acting out of past experiences, current feelings, and future resolutions. By emphasizing sensory systems, emotions, and direct connections to motor action, change is encouraged with less emphasis on the frontal, declarative systems than in other therapies. Primary integration centers seem likely to be highly active during Gestalt therapy experiences, while frontal/hippocampal declarative integration systems seem likely to be less active during intense experiences. Complex neural network patterns are presumed to be activated through implicit connections more than through declarative, explicit decision-making. The resolution of incongruence between declarative awareness and non-declarative, implicit processes unfolds as declarative awareness of implicit processes is facilitated through Gestalt experiences in therapy. Integration of implicit and explicit processing is assumed to lead to the development of explicit decisions that are more effective because they incorporate implicit processing.

The focus on intense experience of events during Gestalt therapies highlights opportunities for activating neural networks from a variety of points of intervention. Each sensory system offers a channel for activating important networks, and enhancement of related emotions likely facilitates recovery of past memories and the various brain systems that compose these memories. Visceral and proprioceptive elements of experiences can also be activated. Motor reenactment incorporates motor systems in the exploration of past learning in ways that other theories do not typically encourage, and taking action offers yet another channel through which old, maladaptive networks can be primed. While minimizing frontal/hippocampal analysis, Gestalt techniques appear to include other brain systems as completely as possible.

Adding consideration of brain function to Gestalt approaches can improve understanding of how specific experiences relate to positive change. Consideration of various modes of input into the brain can foster systematic consideration of ways to heighten a Gestalt experience. Consideration of various channels of output can improve selection of behaviors to encourage during an experience in therapy. Recognition that anxiety is an integral part of experiences supports effective consideration of anxiety as part of the development of new experiences, and can highlight the potential value of anxiety as a guide to the development of complete Gestalt experiences. Acknowledgement of the roles of declarative frontal/hippocampal systems in integrating new knowledge can lead to more effective integration of experiential events into a client's current functioning.

There may be times when conscious examination of how experience can lead to positive change needs to be avoided in order that the connections between maladaptive experiences and positive motor and implicit thought systems can develop without interference from frontal, conscious systems; however, there may be times at which encouraging conscious examination is useful. If a person is experiencing anger with a parent during reenactment of a past event and then is generating alterative responses to that parent, it may be more helpful to allow the client to experience the expression of new responses simultaneously with experiencing the previous event; conscious consideration of declarative rationales for doing this might shift focus away from the connections themselves, thereby weakening the discovery of new procedural connections that could support positive change in the future. Alternatively, it may be helpful to facilitate connection of declarative understanding of the therapeutic experience to the neural networks associated with the events themselves in order that frontal executive decision-making systems can guide conscious use of new learning in future situations. After the client has experienced being more assertive with the parent during reenactment of the memory of the past, conscious choices can be made to apply such changes to current experiences with adults in authority in current life.

Medical interventions

The current framework of overall brain function offers a context within which medical interventions can be conceptualized. Such conceptualization has the potential to foster more complete understanding of the implications of the use of various medications, and can promote more intentional use of medications in coordination with psychotherapeutic intervention as a whole.

Current guidelines for making decisions regarding medication begin with diagnosis and identification of medication-responsive target symptoms associated with the diagnosis. Medications are then typically selected based on empirical findings that have demonstrated positive effects of specific medications on the symptom or pattern (Janicak et al., 2001) (Figure 11.1). This process of decision-making is acknowledged to be less effective than making decisions based on specific understanding of the underlying etiology of the symptom or pattern, and the approach can lead to inappropriate treatment of multiple individual symptoms with multiple medications. However, the level of knowledge in the field precludes more frequent use of etiology in decision-making. Rationales for medication selection are developed in light of connections between symptoms, symptom constellations, diagnoses, neurotransmitters, and the neural pathways within which the individual transmitters have their effects. This approach includes recognition that neural pathways activate specific areas of the brain, and that specific cognitive and emotional activities are mediated by specific areas (Stahl, 2000). However, it does not appear that specific effects on individual cognitive and emotional activities are typically viewed within an overall model of how the brain processes information and generates responses.

Use of medications to manage obsessive compulsive disorder offers an example of the potential benefits of viewing the effects of medication within a broad framework of brain function. Selective Serotonin

Reuptake Inhibitor (SSRI) medications are the current treatments of choice for obsessive compulsive disorder (Janicak *et al.*, 2001). Even though reduction in obsessive symptoms includes disengagement from activities, the possibility that such disengagement could interfere with desirable maintenance of focus during some adaptive, daily activities is often not addressed or is not addressed in depth when considering the potential impact of medication (Janicak *et al.*, 2001; Physicians' Desk Reference, 2003; Stahl, 2000). Active consideration of the potential effects of increasing disengagement tendencies could help the physician and other involved professionals remain alert for possible disruptions in the patient's attention and motivation. If the patient were a student, adults including parents and teachers could be guided to offer extra structure to the student in a positive rather than a punitive way if the potential for increased distractibility could be explained as a side effect of medications needed for management of obsessiveness. Recognition that brain systems that mediate obsessiveness may also affect attention and motivation is likely to result in using medications in more effective ways.

Symptom patterns can be understood in light of the brain systems involved, and this understanding can guide decisions regarding medication. A client's pattern of explosive behavior can be considered in light of the ways various brain systems operate, and the choice of medications can be altered as a result of this consideration. If the patient becomes agitated and explosive in the presence of both positive and negative emotional stimulation, the problem is likely to be the result of poor modulation of brain stem mechanisms controlling overall arousal levels. Medications to manage general arousal might be considered. If the person experiences explosive responses only in the presence of negative emotions, affective dyscontrol might be considered to be the core of the problem, and mood stabilizers might be selected. If the client experiences explosiveness related to a particular issue, such as sadness secondary to abandonment, the clinician would evaluate for the presence of major depression and consider prescribing antidepressant medications. If the client's explosiveness primarily occurs while attempting writing tasks at school, the contribution of a learning disability to distress and emotional reactivity could be identified and addressed in conjunction with medication to manage emotional lability. Identifying particular brain mechanisms involved may contribute to improved decision-making regarding medications to be prescribed.

Consideration of underlying brain processes mediating change in psychotherapy can help determine how to coordinate use of medication in conjunction with psychotherapy. In treating anxiety it may be important that the person's level of anxiety be low enough that they are willing to confront situations that trigger the anxiety. Medication can be used to help the client manage the fear associated with confronting the sources of the fear. However, if the client is taking so much medication that the client has no emotional reaction to the external triggers for fear, one hypothesis would suggest that the person would be unable to habituate to the triggers since habituation requires that the synapses involved be used to the point of depleting the neurotransmitters used for firing, thereby allowing the stimulus neurons to fire without triggering fear. A different brain-based treatment rationale might support elimination of anxiety to the greatest extent possible in order to help build connections between environmental stimuli and new behaviors that can occur in the absence of anxiety. Conceptualizations of the influences of medication on brain functioning can thus guide consideration of when and how much to offer medication to clients dealing with specific issues.

Consideration of the effects of one brain system on another can alter decision-making regarding medications. In the case of deciding whether to offer medication for management of Attention Deficit/Hyperactivity Disorder, a physician might be inclined to delay use of medication as long as the parents feel capable of controlling a child's behaviors without using medications. In this way possible negative side effects could be avoided. However, reduced capacity for attention may interfere significantly with the child's capacity to learn how social interactions work or to learn multi-step academic work. This is particularly important in light of recognition that developmental windows can close (see Chapter 8), since it is possible that lack of adequate attention capacity during the period that a system's window for development is open might result in the system not developing appropriately. Attachment and language systems might both be vulnerable to such a series of events unfolding. In addition, if the decision not to offer medication for problems with attention and impulsivity leads to chronic negative responses by significant adults toward a child, the likelihood is high that the child's positive bonds with others and positive attitudes toward self may be seriously disrupted. Use of stimulant medication in such situations may be important in order to help facilitate the establishment of bonds with others and positive attitudes toward self as secondary benefits of using stimulant medications to improve attention and impulse control.

Summary

The connections outlined thus far between brain functioning and major theories of psychotherapy can now be integrated within the overarching framework presented in the previous chapters of this book. The framework includes details encapsulated in Figures 1.1 and 9.1, along with references to developmental contributions and contrasts between implicit and explicit memory processes.

Intellectual functioning as assessed in traditional intellectual and achievement batteries and in neuropsychological evaluations is not typically included in assessment or intervention in the major schools of psychotherapy, so emphasis on this in the current model adds to assessment and intervention conceptualizations. Behavioral techniques rely on changing implicit connections between incoming stimuli and either direct associations or operant consequences. Gestalt techniques emphasize the activation of implicit systems through sensory input, stimulation of primary integration/neural network connections, and motor expression, with explicit processing being used to intentionally guide this activation; change is conceived to involve integration of declarative and implicit elements in a way that is generated by the client rather than guided by conscious development of new skills. Psychodynamic interventions emphasize the uncovering of implicit memories and the subsequent connection of these memories with declarative processes. Therapist directed explicit, declarative development of new patterns to substitute for old patterns is not part of traditional psychodynamic intervention. Cognitive behavioral techniques that focus on changing irrational thoughts strongly emphasize explicit rather than implicit processes, assuming that changes in implicit processes will occur if changes in explicit processing have occurred. Cognitive-behavioral and behavioral techniques that are focused on skill development rely on explicit systems to help develop new neural networks that can substitute for previously developed maladaptive networks. This explicitly based development of new networks can add to the emphasis on implicit processing systems that characterizes psychodynamic and Gestalt interventions. Cognitive behavioral constructivist approaches appear to integrate activation of implicit systems, resolution of differences in explicit and implicit patterns, and explicit development of new skills. Psychopharmacological interventions have the potential to affect all processing systems, and are viewed as potentially critical contributors to changes involving any element of the framework.

Cognitive assessment, the various schools of psychotherapy, and medical intervention can each offer useful tools and strategies to clinicians and clients during the psychotherapy process. The neuroscience model of intervention presented here recognizes these potential contributions. The neuroscience model may help improve the effectiveness of how each individual model is applied. At the same time, the neuroscience model also offers a context within which strengths of each type of intervention can be more effectively integrated in a coordinated fashion during implementation of psychological therapies.

20

Applying neuroscience to depression intervention

Previous chapters have provided a broad conceptualization of personal functioning relevant to psychotherapy. This conceptualization has been applied to psychological interventions in general, and connections have been identified between the current framework and traditional psychotherapies. The present neuroscience model of psychological therapies can also be used as the framework within which specific diagnoses or syndromes are treated.

Treatment of depression provides an opportunity to demonstrate how a neuroscience approach can be applied to psychological problems identified as part of a specific diagnosis. In this chapter, issues associated with the definition and diagnosis of depression will be discussed in light of a neuroscience approach. Genetic and developmental influences on the expression of depression will be discussed in terms of brain processes. Behaviors, thoughts, and emotions that characterize depression will be tied to brain function, and the treatment implications of brain anatomy and processes will be described. Specific applications of neuropsychological concepts and the concept of neural networks will be delineated. Techniques will be offered for integrating discussion of the brain into discussions with clients regarding depression, and implications of brain function for client improvement will be highlighted. In the course of the discussion of applying neuroscience to the treatment of depression, similarities to and differences from traditional models of intervention with depressed clients will be noted.

Definition of depression

A clear and specific definition of depression remains elusive (Klein *et al.*, 2006; Maj & Sartorius, 1999). Boundaries between depression and other diagnoses and areas of psychological difficulty have been established to only a limited degree, and questions exist regarding variations within the realm of depression itself.

Boundaries between depression and some associated disorders appear to have been well-established, while other boundaries remain hotly debated (Klein *et al.*, 2006). The manic aspect of Bipolar I Disorder has been consistently differentiated from Major Depressive Disorder, but it has not been clearly established whether the depressive aspect of Bipolar I Disorder is the same as or different from depression within Major Depressive Disorder. Connections between depression and anxiety have been both advocated and questioned. The appropriate locations of boundaries between depression and normal responses to grief and loss have also been debated.

Within the diagnosis of Major Depressive Disorder, questions have been raised regarding the existence of discrete subtypes of depression. A recent summary of the field addressed "psychotic depression", "endogenous depression (melancholia)", and "neurotic and reactive depression" as possible concepts useful in considering variations within the diagnosis of depression (Klein *et al.*, 2006). The presence of psychotic features may reflect connection with Bipolar I Disorder, and may be associated with poorer prognosis. Endogenous depression may reflect the presence of a distinct entity within the diagnosis of depression, although it is possible that endogenous depression represents a difference in severity rather than type when contrasted with reactive depression.

Researchers have emphasized that attempts with current diagnostic schema (DSM-IV TR and ICD-10) to define and subcategorize mood disorders based on symptom patterns have been useful, but that, "none of these categories appears to be clearly demarcated from its neighbors" (Kendell, 1999, p. 53). An increasingly accepted view is that depression, as well as other psychiatric disorders, is influenced by a variety of genes (Plomin & McGuffin, 2003) interacting with a variety of environmental influences (Caspi *et al.*, 2003). Following this reasoning, it has been proposed that consideration of the various components of depression can lead to more effective identification of causes, processes, and interventions (Hasler *et al.*, 2004). Furthermore, it has been proposed that early and repeated stressful experiences result in long-term alterations in brain systems that increase vulnerability to the onset of depression (Southwick *et al.*, 2005). Research indicates that repeated episodes of depression contribute to increased sensitivity to progressively milder stressors as well as increasing likelihood that depression can be triggered in the absence of significant identifiable stressors (Monroe & Harkness, 2005).

The neuroscience approach to psychological therapies provides a context within which a therapist can understand the current state of affairs regarding the diagnosis of depression. A neuropsychological approach emphasizes that various types of behavior rely on different underlying brain systems. This conceptualization can be applied just as well to features of depression as it can be to elements of cognitive processing including attention, verbal versus visual-spatial processing, and levels of integration of language. Different symptoms are likely to reflect different disruptions in underlying brain functioning (Hasler *et al.*, 2004). For example, depressed mood may be the result of disruption in serotonin systems while anhedonia may result from dysfunction in brain reward systems mediated by dopamine. Other symptoms discussed in this manner by Hasler and colleagues (2004) include impaired attention and concentration, impaired long-term memory, neurovegetative symptoms, diurnal variations, psychomotor retardation, psychomotor agitation, and increased stress sensitivity. Each symptom of depression can be considered in light of underlying brain structures, transmitters, and transmitter systems that contribute to the expression of the symptom by the patient. Focus on symptoms and constellations of symptoms within the diagnosis of depression can guide the clinician to develop interventions that are most likely to be helpful in light of the specific brain systems that may be involved (Janicak *et al.*, 2001).

Treatment

Treatment of depression following the recommendations included in the overall model of neuroscience model includes several steps. The intake process gathers information about specific depressive symptoms as well as about family history, gestation, early physical development, early social development, social experiences across the lifespan, and other areas of current functioning. Therapy is then implemented in light of the identified areas of strength and weakness. Therapy implementation is designed to influence multiple discrete aspects of brain functioning as discussed in subsequent paragraphs. The conclusion of therapy includes specific considerations outlined in the overall model and discussed below with regard to depression.

This series of steps provides a structure within which neuroscience concepts can guide treatment in at least three ways. First, treatment can be implemented that targets specific brain systems supporting the symptom. Second, treatment can be implemented that avoids reliance on specific brain systems that symptoms suggest are not functioning adequately. Finally, exploring a specific symptom, such as a specific mood or thought pattern, can activate neural networks associated with that symptom. Activation of one network can then lead to activation of related networks, thereby using activation of one brain pattern to lead to subsequent identification of related brain systems and symptoms that suggest effective avenues of treatment.

The Big Picture (Figure 9.1) offers a concrete guide within which depressive functioning and treatment can be considered. Interventions can be designed in light of both trait and state strengths and weaknesses. That is, some characteristics of the client's processing, for example, verbal intelligence, will be present whether the client is depressed or not, while other characteristics of functioning, such as anxiety or depressed mood, may be transient expressions of the client's current depressed state. The client will have a unique cognitive input–process–output pattern on which the client can rely and on which treatment can be based. One client may have strong verbal capacities while another may rely primarily on non-verbal processing of input and generation of output. Anxiety, mood, arousal levels, and patterns of past experience connected to current understanding of life can each contribute to the set of symptoms of depression the client presents. The client's executive functioning including decision-making, attention, impulse control, and reasoning may be impaired due to the depression or due to chronic limitation in a specific process. Identification of strengths and weaknesses prior to the depression as well as at the time of the depression can guide selection of interventions.

Cognitive behavior therapy (CBT) is a primary therapy strategy used in the treatment of depression. Christensen and colleagues (Christensen *et al.*, 2006) described ways that CBT can influence a variety of cognitive deficits that often occur as part of depression. Affected processes identified by these researchers included information-processing speed, psychomotor speed, general attention, attention bias, memory impairment, mood–memory connections, inhibition, automatic cognitive processes, and effortful cognitive processes. They described how CBT interventions can disrupt depressive cognitions through both activation of more positive content and shifting from automatic thoughts to intentional, effortful thinking. Within the current neuroscience approach, the shift would involve increased activation of executive, frontal, explicit memory systems in ways that disrupt implicit processes related to maladaptive ideas and mood. Neural networks that include functioning in all parts of the brain are shifted in ways that begin to activate non-depressive functioning. Arousal levels, anxiety, mood, and patterns associated with previous negative experiences can all be positively activated by such a change in frontal lobe processing, and such changes can then alter the quality of the input–process–output flow of information through the brain during daily experiences.

The Big Picture suggests that CBT interventions focus on one aspect of overall brain functioning in order to change depressed processing throughout the brain. Research supports the effectiveness of this interven-tion, but the present model suggests that viewing depression as involving disruption in multiple areas of the brain would lead to a broader range of interventions that could be applied flexibly to address the symptoms of the individual client. For example, a client experiencing severe slowing in information processing and psychomotor speed would likely be unable to support the cognitive activity required for implementation of CBT interventions. Such a client would be more likely to benefit from interventions designed to influence mood and arousal rather than complex verbal reasoning.

In order to initiate a change in mood and arousal it might be more effective to begin with simple tasks that activate lower levels of the brain while requiring minimal activation of frontal and executive areas of the brain affected by the depression. When changes in mood and arousal are initiated, changes in overall function may follow by way of changes in neural networks that are activated.

The therapist might recommend that the client engage in simple motor tasks such as walking around the block or vacuuming one room in the house. It might also be appropriate to recommend that the client do tasks that are passive but that activate hedonic systems that are shut down at the beginning of treatment. For example, if a client enjoys watching old movies, but typically feels guilty for doing so because of the perception that this "wastes time", it might be helpful to recommend watching the movies since to initiate such an activity requires little ongoing arousal, motivation, positive self-assessment, reduction in anxiety, or change in patterns of perception. Activation of positive neural networks could thereby be achieved with minimal requirement of motivation and effort.

In a different therapeutic situation, the therapist could ask the client to recall a previous positive experience, and then use the session to guide the client to full experiencing of that memory. The appropriateness of such an intervention would be highest if the therapist had previously heard the client describe such an event, since the therapist's knowledge of relatively recent activation of such a memory would let the therapist know that the likelihood of successful recall of the positive event is high. The therapist could ask the client to describe multiple sensory elements of the experience, describe the mood associated with the various elements of the experience, and describe interpersonal activities associated with the experience. The client might not be asked to consciously contrast that experience with the current depressive state, since such frontal cognitive activity is conceived to disengage the client from lower level channels of brain activity that have been "opened" by simply elaborating the neural networks associated with previous positive experience. For one client, recalling the previous, positive experience may, by itself, be enough to initiate a shift in brain processing, while for another client, challenging self-statements may initiate change more effectively. In either case there has been an increase in activity level in networks associated with non-depressive overall brain functioning.

If anxiety was identified as a prominent element of the depressive episode, interventions to manage anxiety could be initiated. Diaphragmatic breathing is a basic strategy that requires relatively little practice before results are obtained. More elaborate progressive relaxation training using repetitions of tensing and releasing muscle groups requires higher levels of effort and motivation than basic breathing techniques, but progressive relaxation relies on concrete behaviors rather than abstract thoughts, and can therefore be more easily enacted for some clients than can changes in logical verbal statements. The relaxed state achieved through the use of relaxation techniques can begin to disrupt the extant pattern of functioning that keeps a depressed client from making progress. If the client has experienced anxiety while initiating activities that provoke guilt, reducing the anxiety may allow the client to recognize how guilt interferes, and new choices in behavior can then be made. If a previously mentioned client felt guilty for watching movies, anxiety may have preceded participation in such guilt-inducing activities and may have contributed to blocking the activity. Relaxation could help change this. In addition, taking active steps to learn relaxation is likely to activate neural networks that include relevant brain systems that are associated with being an active and successful person, and such networks can then help dislodge the depression. Furthermore, receiving support from the therapist during the development of relaxation skills can activate networks associated with being cared for and bonded with another person, and neural networks associated with these experiences can help the client move out of the depressed state.

While symptoms of depression are often viewed as problems to be corrected, it may also be useful to treat symptoms of depression as clues to be explored. Since the client is already mired in depression, activation of depressed neural networks would not require high levels of arousal, frontal inhibition and initiation processes, and activation of competing networks. The therapist could suggest to the client that exploring neural networks associated with the depression might lead to an understanding that can guide future change. The client would be encouraged to focus on the current mood and then to notice what pops into the client's head. If a specific image or memory emerged for the client, the therapist would then help the client elaborate the memory by asking about associated sensations, thoughts, motor behaviors, and emotions. Identifying and elaborating neural networks could lead to recognition of triggers for the current depression, which could then allow changes in cognitive appraisal from global to specific, a central goal in CBT. Such identification could also reveal potential positive networks that could be activated in order to dislodge the depression.

Exploration of depressive neural networks might result in failure to identify specific memories or images that could lead to change. However, from the beginning of such an exploration of connections with the depressed mood the therapist would frame the exploration as only one avenue of possible change, thereby keeping expectations realistic and reducing the potential for emotional disappointment. In addition, even though the content of the exploration has not seemed useful, the process of working actively and intentionally with the caring therapist may activate networks associated with frontal, intentional functioning and with feeling emotionally connected rather than abandoned. Neural networks associated with positive functioning might then be more likely to become active in the future.

As with other therapeutic interventions, psychopharmacological treatments vary in their effects on different elements of brain functioning and can therefore be selected based on symptom patterns that reflect specific patterns of brain activity (Hasler et al., 2004). Selective serotonin reuptake inhibitors are considered to influence mood as well as frontal lobe brain systems associated with executive processing. Medications that influence norepinephrine and dopamine systems may affect reward systems and hedonic aspects of depression. If anxiety is a prominent aspect of depression, benzodiazepines may be useful (Janicak et al., 2001). Mechanisms other than neurotransmitter activity have been identified as likely to influence the presence or absence of depression, and medications that influence various neuronal processes in disparate areas of the brain likely differentially affect specific symptoms of depression. It is not possible in the present venue to review all potential disruptions and all potential psychopharmacological interventions. Rather, in the present context it is important to maintain awareness that activity within neurons, between neurons, and in systems of neurons throughout the brain can be influenced by medications in ways that account for activity in specific areas of the brain and for related observable symptoms. Psychopharmacological intervention for depression can be considered as one of many interventions that target unique brain activity associated with unique symptom patterns.

The conclusion of therapy for depression may involve helping the client return to previous levels of adaptive functioning or may require the development of new skills and patterns to substitute for previous chronic patterns that have contributed in the past to vulnerability to the onset of depression. In either case, dealing with improvement as well as with the maintenance of success is likely to be important.

If the patient has a long history of successful functioning in many areas of life, recovery from depression is less likely to trigger anxiety associated with novelty as described in Chapter 16. However, such a patient should be explicitly told that stress, anxiety, and depressed mood are all likely to occur in the future as part of normal functioning. This can help reduce the possibility that panic occurs in reaction to minor symptoms. The patient should be guided to consider the application of specific coping strategies to normal events and to the initial mild symptoms of depression that may occur at times. Such a review at a time when the client is coping well is assumed to establish a connection between intervention strategies and possible symptoms at the same time that positive neural networks are active. It is hoped that future experience of minor symptoms can be connected to positive mood and a sense of self-efficacy, and the negative effects of such symptoms can thereby be reduced. Finally, symptoms that warrant return to treatment could be identified, thereby increasing the possibility that the patient will return to treatment before a return of depression becomes overwhelming.

If the patient has a long history of poor adaptive functioning, it is likely that improvement during treatment will itself trigger distress and confusion that may be experienced by the patient (or the therapist) as signs of regression during treatment. Following guidelines offered in Chapter 16, it can be explained to the patient that anxiety associated with unfamiliar positive functioning is likely due to the novelty of the experience as well as to the lack of neural networks associated with positive functioning. This explanation can support reduction in anxiety and maintenance of hopefulness that improvement is occurring. It will then be important to help the patient develop skills and patterns of adaptive responding to use in the future. It may be critical to help the patient develop social skills, relaxation strategies, lists of activities from which to derive enjoyment, and adaptive approaches to experiencing relationships. It is expected that development of neural networks associated with each of these types of functioning will reduce the likelihood that depression will recur.

Concepts of brain function

The current neuroscience approach to describing and treating different versions of depression has multiple implications. Each implication influences the approaches clinicians take during interventions to help ameliorate depression.

Each version of depression is considered to be a collection of activities distributed throughout the brain. The neural network concept captures the essence of this view. Interventions that alter function in any one area may shift functioning in others. However, no one area of activity is considered to be the "core" of depression. This conceptualization is consistent with the multi-gene view of the heritability of depression (Plomin & McGuffin, 2003), and is consistent with the gene-by-experience-interaction view of the expression of depressive symptoms (Caspi *et al.*, 2003). Thus, CBT focused on changing self-talk may be effective in ameliorating depression, but this does not mean that depression is primarily a "disorder of self-statements". Rather, various interventions that each uniquely affects a specific aspect of depressive function may positively affect a given version of depression. The current conceptualization encourages a whole-brain view of depression and promotes consideration of a variety of types of intervention, depending on the specific symptoms identified.

One characteristic of the "collection of brain activities" view is that it incorporates trait as well as state features of functioning. It may be that a client processes information almost completely through non-verbal channels rather than verbal ones. This is not due to depression, but it profoundly influences the pattern of symptoms and the avenues through which psychotherapy can effect change. For such a client, activities rather than verbal self-statements would need to be the medium of intervention. In order to increase the client's likelihood of viewing negative events as time limited rather all-encompassing, a combination of drawings and time-lines might be a more effective intervention than talking about the global and specific aspects of specific events.

Residual effects of early trauma may also be considered to be trait rather than state characteristics of depression. For example, there is substantial evidence that early trauma negatively affects hippocampal size (Ford, 2005), and the implication would be that the capacity for integrative thinking would be impaired as a result of such events. For a client affected by such early events, learning steps of positive interventions might be more appropriate than developing an in-depth conceptualization of issues related to the experience of depression.

Each version of depression is viewed as consisting of discrete elements, and each element calls for interventions designed to influence that element. Conscious self-talk is likely to be influenced by the development of strategies to identify and alter maladaptive thoughts. Psychomotor slowing and/or severe reduction in information processing may best be addressed through prescription of very simple behaviors that initially require low levels of effort. Reduced ability to find a sense of reward through activity may benefit from the development of basic self-gratifying behaviors that can support subsequent activity in various realms of a person's life. A unique set of interventions used can be chosen for use with each client in light of the symptoms demonstrated rather than due to the diagnosis of the presence of depression.

The potential for specific psychotherapeutic interventions to effectively influence specific symptoms and associated underlying brain systems is likely to change over the course of treatment. A severely depressed patient with low energy, anhedonia, and negative self-talk may initially not be able to respond to traditional CBT interventions. The patient may only be able to effectively undertake CBT interventions after simpler interventions can be completed that result in an increase in the patient's energy level and speed of information processing. Interventions to improve energy level might include initiation of simple physical activities such as walking the dog, or might consist of psychopharmacological treatment. The various elements of depressive functioning may thus best be served by a series of interventions that depend on the unique trait and state patterns characterizing the client and his depression at specific moments in the therapy process. No one intervention is considered to be the primary treatment; rather each is critical for intervention leading to the development of successful brain function.

There is a corollary to the admonition to treat the symptom that is available for successful intervention: work around areas of functioning that are not amenable to direct intervention. This was implied in the earlier discussion of developing strategies for treating a client whose non-verbal abilities are stronger than verbal abilities. It is proposed that by working around the deficit in verbal processing, change in depressive functioning throughout the brain can be effected even though verbal self-statements cannot be directly addressed.

In a somewhat similar situation, there may be psychological issues that overwhelm the client, and that may therefore need to be avoided for a time during therapy. If a client is overwhelmed by memories related to past abuse, it may be useful to help the client explore depressive cognitions in contexts outside the realm of abuse. It may be that the current depression will remit without full exploration of the abuse, or it may be that as the client gains psychological strength and stamina through reduction of depression, the client will become capable of successfully processing past abuse so that the client is less likely to be overwhelmed by life experiences in the future.

Focus on symptoms rather than diagnosis guides the therapist and the client to focus on relevant areas of difficulty that may not be part of the diagnosis of depression. For example, discussions during the course of treatment may reveal the presence of a long-standing problem with social relatedness that reflects the presence of a mild version of Asperger's Disorder characterized by significant difficulty understanding social interactions and relationships. Appropriate treatment would include development of conscious awareness of patterns of social interaction accompanied by recognition of and ability to use appropriate behaviors in social situations. Similarly, it might become evident during treatment that problems with attention and concentration have been present at times when the client was not experiencing depression. It would then be important to develop interventions that could help the client maintain optimal attention and concentration while also developing strategies to offset weakness in this area. The client might be encouraged to sit at the front of any meeting, always carry a calendar for scheduling, and develop a daily routine that includes checking the calendar. Both these instances are conceived as including identification of symptoms that would not be identified if rigid focus was maintained on behaviors comprising depression.

Interventions designed to reduce specific symptoms of depression can be understood within a neuroscience framework to stimulate changes not related to the content of the intervention. It has been proposed that separate systems exist for taking positive action and for avoiding problems (Derryberry & Tucker, 1992). Often depression includes being inactive, and the process of taking any active step toward recovery may activate systems that can support active coping rather than passive avoidance. Getting off the couch to choose and then insert a movie from the client's video collection may stimulate systems associated with active coping even though the physical action of starting the movie is itself small.

Another example of inadvertent change is tied to unintentional triggering of neural networks underlying past experiences. Most treatment interventions activate a pattern that includes the client being helped to cope with difficulties in life. This may activate transference reactions that either support or interfere with the implementation of therapy. If receiving help is acceptable to client, the helping context of treatment can lead to greater feelings of safety and well-being, and these feelings may purposely or inadvertently support the implementation of the planned treatment. However, if the experience of needing and feeling gratified by receiving help threatens the client's sense of security, negative reactions may undermine the process of treatment.

Discussing the brain and depression with the client

An important benefit of a neuroscience approach to psychotherapy of depression is that it offers both a context and an understandable language within which the client can be helped to view the disorder and treatment. This concept was discussed in a general way in Chapter 18 (see Table 18.1), but it is worth considering in the context of a specific disorder.

Explanations of the neuroscience of depression offer clear, concrete explanations for the emotions, thoughts, and behaviors clients experience.

This is particularly relevant to the treatment of depression since problems with low mood, low energy, slowed thinking, and difficulty concentrating are frequently experienced as coming "out of the blue" while they simultaneously interfere with positive cognitive re-conceptualization. A client often cannot see why symptoms of depression have emerged, so there is a tendency to assume the symptoms of depression are expressions of the core of the person. This problem is further exacerbated by the tendency for negative mood to trigger negative memories and ideas that are congruent with the depression. Identifying elements of depression and the brain systems that support them can help turn all symptoms into problems to be solved rather than negative characteristics of the self. The elementary diagram of brain functioning (Figure 1.1) and the Big Picture (Figure 9.1) can be used during discussions to guide this re-conceptualization. Discussion of interactions between different elements, including identification of strengths and weaknesses in the different areas of functioning, encourages clients to recognize that seemingly intractable symptoms may be led to change.

Understanding the neuroscience underpinnings of depression helps clients participate in interventions that may lead to change. A depressed client being asked to recall in detail a previous positive experience was observed to argue with such an instruction on the basis of the client's belief that the experience did not fit the way things "really are". That is, the previous positive experience was inconsistent with the client's current depressive perception of the world. The same client was observed to cooperate with the intervention when it was pointed out that the client need not alter the current conscious cognitive assessment of the event. It was explained that the memory to be activated was already part of the client's repertoire, it was not necessary to identify it as reasonable or not, and it might activate more positive elements of functioning through activation of positive neural networks. The client's conscious cognitions regarding the situation subsequently shifted in a positive direction after she was helped to immerse herself in the memory of the previous positive experience. This shift occurred despite the absence of direct attempts to alter the client's negative cognitions.

Responses to recommendations for medication have similarly been observed to be more positive when offered in conjunction with explanations regarding which brain systems are likely to change in what ways in order to lead to what specific changes in depression. Discussing medication for depression in such a way reduces the extent to which taking medication seems like a moral failure. Such discussion also allows the client to begin to perceive medication as changing specific elements of functioning rather than changing the whole person.

Conclusion

Neuroscience concepts appear to have great potential to improve the diagnosis of depression, or rather, the diagnosis of the various symptoms that reflect underlying brain functioning that leads to the experience of depressive symptoms. Viewing depression as a collection of various interwoven elements from cellular to brain system to behavioral levels can guide development of treatment strategies, implementation of specific interventions, and communication with the client throughout the treatment process. Finally, application of neuroscience concepts to the treatment of depression offers one clear example of how applying neuroscience to psychological therapies can lead to improved treatment.

21

Neuroscience and psychotherapy: moving forward

Brain science at its current level of development offers enough facts to support a new way of approaching psychotherapy. This seems true even though the quality of the data available is not yet adequate to qualify brain-based psychotherapy as "empirically based" intervention. Despite the absence of clinical outcome research to support brain-based interventions, the neuroscience approach can positively influence theoretical conceptualization of the process of psychotherapy as well as immediate clinical application.

A framework for understanding brain processes related to psychotherapy was outlined in Part 1 of this book. Neuropsychologically based consideration of input, processing, and output of information by clients helps clarify the ways clients process experiences, and neuropsychological understanding of brain processes can thereby help identify the best means for guiding clients toward positive change. A richer and more complete understanding of how clients process and respond to their experiences in life is derived from recognition of levels of processing ranging from lower brain general arousal systems to mid-brain affective processing to higher cortical cognition; this understanding is enhanced by simultaneous recognition of the various ways each of these levels influences the others. The overarching concept of neural networks ties together the various systems managing information and behavior throughout the brain. The concept of neural networks suggests how past and present experiences are connected and how new, more adaptive connections can be developed. Constant consideration of declarative versus procedural, explicit versus implicit memory systems increases consciousness of how previously developed maladaptive behavior patterns are maintained, how change can occur, and how painfully out of synchrony changes in various parts of the brain can be. Change and failure to change become more understandable and less threatening when these differences in forms of memory are kept in mind. Interpreting emotions as rich sources of information about the self rather than as tools for measuring moral quality can allow clients' responses to their own emotions to become more accepting and more adaptive. Identifying different roles for anxiety in dealing with previously threatening as well as novel stimuli contributes to improved initial exploration of problems, to better management of anxiety when it occurs, and to steadier completion of change undertaken in psychotherapy even though anxiety is likely to recur at various times. Integration of concepts of brain development into understanding of interventions with children and adults results in changes in approach that have the potential to make medical as well as psychotherapeutic interventions more effective.

Part 2 of this book examines implications for specific aspects of psychotherapy implementation. Assessment, conceptualization, intervention, and communication in therapy all seem likely to improve when the underlying nature of brain functioning as currently understood is kept in mind during the implementation of psychotherapy. Consideration of psychotherapy in terms of the framework of brain function offers the potential for integrating and coordinating various traditional treatment modalities within a structure that can facilitate communication between proponents of various schools of treatment, and can support collaborative rather than competitive interventions.

The framework offered in the current book can serve as a context within which deep study as well as broad exploration and application can take place. Studies of "use dependent synaptic plasticity" in a sea slug are deep in more than the underwater sense, focusing as they do on individual connections between neurons as well as on the intraneuronal chemical cascades that bring about synaptic changes. At the same time, implications of this research are far reaching when evaluated within the broad context of the neuroscience of personal and interpersonal functioning. Viewed in such a broad context, results of research with the sea slug suggest reasons for the devastation caused by physical and sexual abuse while also suggesting ways psychological treatment may affect the neural systems of victims. The same studies of the sea slug neural system imply that consistency and repetition in parenting are important for development of the physiological underpinnings of attachment in procedural memory systems of human infants. Viewing human functioning generally and the process of psychotherapy in particular within the context of a neural science framework can facilitate recognition of the multiple implications of any results of neuroscience research.

New information can be considered with regard to its place in the input–process–output flow of information through the brain. It can be considered with regard to influences on declarative as well as procedural memory and processing systems. It can be viewed in light of its place in and influence upon brain development. New knowledge in neuroscience can be interpreted with regard to its influence on internal experiences within clients and with regard to its impact on interactions between clients and surrounding culture. The current framework and set of specific information offer an example of how to integrate new neuroscience findings into the realm of clinical intervention.

In addition to offering a variety of clear implications for explicit conceptualization and intervention, considering the brain as the heart of psychotherapy seems likely to improve clinical intuition rather than to break down psychotherapy into a brain-based mechanistic consideration of clients. Consideration of each element of brain functioning in the processing of an event promotes openness to previously unidentified connections with other parts of the brain rather than fostering constricted focus on the next behaviorally face-valid connection. An element of visual image can trigger emotion, other senses, arousal, conscious cognition, and motor behavior. When therapy is flowing easily, such connections are often integrated without explicit consideration in ways that foster positive change. But when therapy is mired and unmoving, taking time to conceive of elements of brain functioning that are known and then to purposefully allow the potential connections with other aspects of brain functioning to pop into mind can lead to novel considerations that are anchored in how the client's brain really works.

Empathy and communication of understanding appear to be supported by psychotherapy of the brain. Recognition and overt description of the control affect has over the ideas a client diagnosed with borderline personality disorder can conceive or remember can be soothing to the client even when the client continues to have difficulty recalling alternate positive views of self or situation. Clients are soothed by the therapist's expression of understanding and appreciation of the distress experienced when procedural memories are provoking maladaptive behaviors and verbalizations even in the presence of clients' declarative awareness of the irrationality of their responses.

Consideration of the brain increases the therapist's and then the client's appreciation of the subtleties of influence running throughout experience. Mood influences what thoughts pop into a client's awareness when decision-making is being undertaken, so that rational problem-solving can be undermined without the client's awareness. Lowered arousal influences will and determination in trying to carry out goals that have been established during the psychotherapy session. Recognition of these and other characteristics of brain functioning can be used to uphold morale through the slow process of changing the influence of identified and unidentified maladaptive patterns of function. At the same time, failure to succeed in self-control becomes less a sign of moral inadequacy and more a piece of evidence regarding what the brain is doing now and what the client might choose as goals for the future.

The structure and details outlined in this book have the potential to operate beyond themselves. Each reader is likely to bring to the current reading as well as to future reflections a fund of knowledge beyond what is presented here. The expertise may be in a particular form of clinical intervention, in a certain clinical research track or in a specific area of neuroscience research. The knowledge may derive from research not yet completed. In any case, the current outline presents an approach for incorporating new neuroscience information at the same time that it offers a specific framework and a set of evidence that can stand alone.

This presentation of a model of psychotherapy based on understanding of the brain is a beginning. It is rife with weakness in empirical support for ideas proposed. However, it seems that the amount and quality of information available in numerous fields dedicated to understanding brain functioning can support these initial conceptualizations adequately enough to foster some improvements in current implementation of psychotherapy while simultaneously offering a heuristic framework that can encourage more rapid development of related and better supported proposals in the future.

Neuroimaging and psychological therapies

The framework outlined in this book emphasizes two primary concepts related to the interface between the brain and psychological therapies. First, information is processed by way of a series of brain events characterized by an input–process–output flow of activity (see Chapter 2). This concept emphasizes that specific elements of brain processing are carried out in consecutive order, and that specific elements are carried out in specific locations throughout the brain. Second, each experience is based on a unique combination of neural activities that take place throughout the brain (see Chapter 3). This second concept emphasizes that specific structures throughout the brain participating in an experience must be identified in order to understand connections between the brain, personal experience, and psychological therapies. Newly developed imaging techniques used to observe the structures and functions of the brain have shaped the development of this framework for understanding the brain–psychological intervention interface.

Understanding the neuroimaging procedures that are primary sources of hypotheses regarding brain–behavior relationships on which the current framework is based can help the reader to recognize the vast amount that is known about brain function. Simultaneously, awareness of neuroimaging procedures can help the reader to appreciate the significant limitations inherent in each technology on which our knowledge of the brain is based. Finally, basic understanding of neuroimaging techniques that are increasingly the primary foundation for understanding the brain–behavior interface can help the reader assess research results more realistically and integrate them into the current framework more effectively.

This appendix will first describe general concepts related to neuroimaging strategies as a whole. Individual neuroimaging techniques will then be briefly described along with examples of the use of specific techniques to provide information incorporated into the framework of neuroscience and psychological therapies. Research strategies combining the varying strengths of the different imaging tools will be described. Finally, implications for future understanding of processes related to psychological therapies will be discussed.

It is important to note what the current review will and will not do. It will offer a brief overview of the most prominent neuroimaging techniques currently in use in research and clinical applications. It will direct the reader to resources offering moderately complex descriptions of individual technologies. The current review will offer clinically relevant examples of the ways in which individual technologies impact under-standing of interactions between the brain and clinical interventions. The current review will not offer in-depth descriptions of the technologies involved, although it seems clear that the greater the reader's understanding of the technologies involved, the better will be the reader's ability to apply research findings to the clinical field. The current review will not provide exhaustive descriptions of neuroimaging research results relevant to clinical intervention. This book as a whole is designed to establish for the reader a starting point from which the reader can explore and apply myriad findings in many fields within the domain of neuroscience. Similarly, this Appendix is designed to offer a basic starting point from which neuroimaging techniques can be explored in greater detail.

Neuroimaging techniques: general concepts

The first computed tomography (CT) images produced in the late 1960s opened a window into the brain that had previously not existed. The first implementation of CT technology allowed researchers as well as clinicians to view brain structures without the disruptive intrusions of surgery or... death. Since that time, a variety of technologically complex tools for unintrusively examining brain structure and function have been developed. These include positron emission tomography (PET), single photon emission computed tomography (SPECT), magnetic resonance imaging (MRI), and functional magnetic resonance imaging (fMRI) (Dougherty et al., 2004). In addition, electroencephalography (EEG), which provides an overall assessment of brain activity, seems appropriate to consider along with these other techniques even though it does not yield a neuroimage of the brain that is similar to the brain's physical contours.

A primary feature of the neuroimaging techniques (but not EEG) is that they provide a three-dimensional representation of the brain. Image information is collected along three separate axes in space and then integrated using computer programs to yield the three-dimensional data field upon which subsequent analyses depend (see Figure A.1). Visual images offered to represent the various

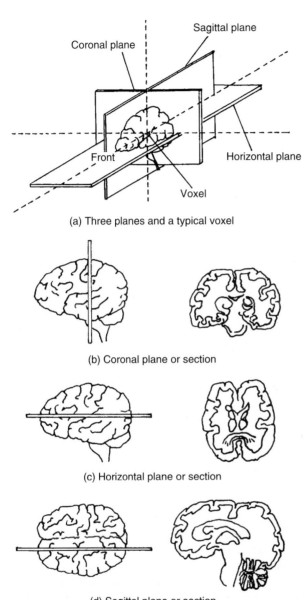

(a) Three planes and a typical voxel

(b) Coronal plane or section

(c) Horizontal plane or section

(d) Sagittal plane or section

Figure A.1 Neuroimages and the brain. A. Representation of three primary orientations of planes or "sections" used in neuroimaging; the "voxel" is the intersection of the planes. B. Coronal plane or section viewed from the front of the brain. C. Horizontal plane or section viewed from above or below the brain. D. Sagittal plane or section viewed from the side.

scans can be presented in the form of a three-dimensional picture of the brain, or in the form of individual "slices" of data on various two-dimensional planes represented as cross-sectional images reflecting structure or activity in the brain in that plane of examination. The two-dimensional images typically present views as if the observer is in front of the subject looking at the brain (coronal section), below the subject looking up at the brain with the person's face at the top of the view (horizontal section), or beside of the person looking at the side of the person's brain (sagittal section) (Saper *et al.*, 2000). Visual images may variously consist of a three-dimensional representation, two-dimensional representations of slices viewed from the front, side, or bottom of the brain, or two-dimensional images along a unique plane of interest.

At least as important as the intriguing visual images provided by neuroimaging techniques is the fact that each specific brain location in three dimensional space is coded within associated computer programs in ways that make that individual space, called a voxel (see Figure A.1), available to a variety of statistical analyses that facilitate interpretation of patterns of data. Such analyses can be conducted using voxels or groups of voxels considered likely to be related to cognitions or behaviors of interest. Once scores are obtained, they can be adjusted (using computer programs) to match the shape of a standard, comparison brain. These adjustments allow scores from a specific area of one brain to be combined with or compared to scores obtained from the same area of other brains. Statistical analyses can then be used to compare the values obtained regarding the area of interest in the brain being scanned to the same brain at other times or to norms previously established for that area of the brain. Scores from brains of a group of subjects identified as the experimental group can be combined and then compared to brains of a group of subjects identified as a normal, control group.

Characteristics of each imaging technique influence the specificity and type of information that can be gathered using the various techniques. Two primary constraints on information that can be gathered are spatial resolution and temporal resolution (for graphic representations of spatial and temporal constraints on the various imaging techniques, see Posner & Raichle, 1994, p. 24, and Huettel *et al.*, 2004, p. 10). At the present time none of the non-invasive neuroimaging techniques used with living brains has a spatial resolution capable of providing information regarding function or structure of individual synapses or neurons. Considered in terms of numbers, the most sensitive neuroimaging techniques have spatial resolutions of slightly less than 1 mm. In contrast, the cell bodies of human neurons range from .00005 to .00012 mm in diameter. Thus, all neuroimaging information reflects the activity of groups of neurons. Electrophysiological techniques such as the EEG have high enough temporal sensitivity to provide information regarding the order of firing of neurons during brain processes, but other techniques are significantly less sensitive. However, the number of neurons required to generate a recordable, functionally relevant electrical field at the surface of the brain is extremely high, so EEG recording is of activity in relatively large groups of neurons rather than in single neurons. Finally, different neuroimaging technologies permit assessment of different aspects of neural functioning, each of which will be addressed in the discussion of the individual technique.

While interpreting and applying findings obtained using any neuroimaging technique, it is critical to keep in mind that these techniques do not allow us to watch neurons in action. This is true even though the brightly colored, clearly labeled images of the brain in action tempt readers to assume they are looking at the brain in action. Instead, each technique assesses a physical phenomenon assumed, based on previous research, to be correlated with brain functioning (Huettel *et al.*, 2004). EEG recordings assess the electrical field generated during brain activity. PET and SPECT images rely on the measurement of radioactive decay of artificially introduced chemical elements thought to attach to specific locations in the brain during neural activity. MRI studies rely on the variations in magnetic fields that characterize different chemical elements in the brain, especially hydrogen. fMRI studies monitor magnetic changes related to blood flow that is assumed to increase during activity in a specific area of the brain. For each of the techniques just mentioned, data generated may not accurately represent the neural process that is supposedly being studied. Maintaining awareness of the assumptions underlying the imaging techniques being used can help the reader appreciate the new information being offered while also helping maintain an appropriate level of skepticism regarding the results being described.

Each neuroimaging technique will be briefly described in order to help the reader understand the types of information obtained using each technique. The two primary static imaging tools (CT and MRI) will be discussed first, followed by discussions of tools used to assess function (EEG, PET, SPECT, and fMRI). Uses, strengths, and weaknesses of each technique will be summarized. Once the individual techniques are described, the strategy of integrating techniques will be outlined, since developing research protocols that allow the strengths of the various techniques to complement each other has contributed substantially to improvements in understanding brain function.

Computed tomography (CT)/computerized axial tomography (CAT)

Computed tomography applies X-ray technology to imaging the brain. An X-ray source transmits gamma rays through the brain and different types of tissue in the brain absorb different amounts of radiation as the rays pass through the brain. The amount of radiation that passes through the brain is measured on the far side of the brain, displaying the shapes of different tissues in the slice or plane through which the X-ray passed. Slices are collected from various two dimensional planes or slices through the brain. Then, computer-assisted algorithms translate the information into three-dimensional units (voxels) that can be analyzed to produce images of the brain at a variety of cross-sectional planes.

CT scans produce static images of the structure of the brain. As a result, they can assess the shapes and sizes of tissues in the brain, and can help identify physical damage to the brain. They do not measure activity in the brain. Voxels can be slightly smaller than $1\,\text{mm}^3$, which is smaller than voxels generated by other static measures of brain structure, such as the MRI. Due to the significant level of radiation exposure entailed in completing CT scans, CT scans are limited in regard to obtaining repeated measures. CT scans have been used to identify volume loss and structural abnormalities in specific areas of the brain in association with schizophrenia, obsessive-compulsive disorder, Alzheimer's disease, and anorexia nervosa, among others (Park & Gonzalez, 2004).

Magnetic resonance imaging (MRI)

Magnetic resonance imaging is based on the fact that different tissues in the brain have different magnetic properties that can be systematically altered in order to help identify structures within the brain. A powerful magnetic field is generated around the brain using a large external magnet, and hydrogen atoms present in amounts that differ across various tissues of the brain become magnetically aligned. Then, brief pulses of radio frequency energy are sent through the brain. These pulses alter the orientation of the magnetically organized hydrogen atoms in ways that vary from tissue type to tissue type. These alterations are measured from several angles, yielding a three-dimensional representation of the brain. As with CT scans, MRI measurements can be organized into individual voxels, and information regarding these voxels can be analyzed to create two-dimensional and three-dimensional representations of the brain.

MRI scans produce static images of the structure of the brain. Voxels generated by MRI can be as small as $1\,\text{mm}^3$, depending on the power of the machinery and the strength of the magnetic field generated. The magnetic and radio frequency elements of the MRI technique do not have the negative physiological effects of repeated exposure to X-ray radiation that are associated with CT technology and, as a result, repeated images can be made over time with no negative effects on subjects. This has permitted repeated imaging of brains over the course of a specific illness or over the course of a lifetime of normal development (Durston *et al.*, 2001). Physiological properties of the MRI procedure allow a variety of scanning procedures and types of data analysis (Goldstein & Price, 2004). These procedures and analyses support the examination of structural features associated with a variety of brain characteristics and anomalies. Examples of brain phenomena examined using variations of MRI technology include normal anatomy, variations in size of individual brain structures, brain hemorrhaging, ischemic blood vessel blockages, edema, brain atrophy, white matter lesions, and demyelination. MRI studies have been used to evaluate alterations in brain structure secondary to early childhood abuse (De Bellis, 2001).

Electroencephalography (EEG)

Electroencephalography measures electrical fields on the surface of the brain associated with excitatory and inhibitory activity in groups of neurons in various parts of the brain. The electrical fields are produced by changes in electrical state within the brain. While CT and MRI scans provide structural images, EEG and other imaging techniques to be discussed shortly provide measures of brain activity. EEG is not sensitive enough to measure activity of a single neuron; rather, it measures electrical fields generated by groups of neurons acting simultaneously. The electrical fields measured are not tied to the actual "firing" of neurons as they reach their action potential. Rather, the fields are generated by the coordinated development of excitatory and inhibitory electrical states within groups of neurons. The excitatory and inhibitory states develop in response to input from other neurons that have fired after reaching their action potential (Westbrook, 2000). Data is collected by a grid of electrodes attached at specified locations across the surface of the scalp, and computerized comparisons between measurements obtained from the different electrodes allow determination of activity levels in different areas of the brain.

EEG recordings provide indications of changes in brain activity over time. EEG recordings are sensitive to changes in activity in milliseconds (thousandths of a second), while other techniques for recording activity range in sensitivity from nine-tenths of a second (fMRI) to 40 seconds (PET) (Posner & Raichle, 1994). EEG thus provides a better assessment of changes in activity over time than most of the various neuroimaging techniques. However, the spatial resolution of EEG recordings, about 6 cm, is much larger than the resolution supported by fMRI, about 2 mm, which means that even though EEG can effectively establish when activities occur, it does a poor job of identifying what areas of the brain contribute to the processes being monitored (Huettel *et al.*, 2004). EEG studies have been used to examine alertness, cognition, memory (Berka *et al.*, 2004), learning, sleep, epilepsy, dementia, and delirium (Kuperberg, 2004). EEG has been used to provide fine-grained temporal analysis of steps of a variety of types of cognitive activity (Posner & Raichle, 1994) and to provide indications of cognitive activity associated with states such as worrying (Carter *et al.*, 1986).

The event related potential (ERP) technique is a variation in the use of EEG technology that allows improved clarity of identification of brain activity over time. A specific stimulus pattern is presented multiple times, and the pattern of EEG response is averaged over time to eliminate random elements that would obscure patterns in a single recording (Kuperberg, 2004). The pattern of brain activation over the time associated with completion of identified processes can then be identified. Examination of ERP patterns helps identify stages of processing as well as length of time from initial stimulus exposure to onset of processing. Strengths and weaknesses with regard to EEG temporal and spatial specificity also apply to ERP analyses. ERP studies have been used to examine language processes, memory, executive functioning, facial perception, and attention, among others (Huettel *et al.*, 2004).

Positron emission tomography (PET)

Positron emission tomography involves the introduction of radioactive material into the brain followed by recording of the output associated with radioactive decay of the material. Radioactive materials used are modifications (called isotopes) of chemicals ordinarily used by the brain during activity (for example, oxygen) and, because of their similarity to elements ordinarily used by the brain during functioning, the radioactive isotopes are carried to locations in the brain in which the materials are used as part of neural activity. Radioactive chemicals can be introduced that subsequently offer indications of regional blood flow, glucose metabolism, or binding of neuroreceptors. Each of these activities is considered to be associated in some way with neural activity. However, it is important to keep in mind that PET images reflect these activities rather than offering direct observation of neuronal activity, and questions remain regarding the nature of ties between actions such as blood flow and the actual process whereby the neurons carry out their work. After the isotope has had time to reach the area of the brain in which it participates in brain activity, the decay is monitored using a camera that identifies the location of the source of the radiation. The more a specific area of the brain uses the radioactive chemical while carrying out a brain activity, the greater the concentration of radioactive signals associated with this activity.

The steps from initial creation of the isotope to measurement by the camera surrounding the area of the body to be studied affect the nature and quality of the PET images that can be obtained related to a specific brain function. The radioactive versions of frequently used chemicals are created in an on-site cyclotron and then typically injected into the blood stream of the subject. The blood stream carries the isotope to the location in the brain in which it is used, and the PET camera then begins to monitor signs of decay that reflect where the chemical is being used. As the radioactive chemical decays it produces a positron which leaves the site of decay and then collides with an electron in nearby tissue, thereby triggering the release of two gamma photons that move in opposite directions out of the brain. The collision resulting in the release of the two gamma photons can occur several millimeters from the site where the chemical is being used by the brain. The camera, which surrounds the brain, records each instance in which gamma photons moving in opposite directions are detected, and uses this simultaneous recording process to identify the location at which the collision between the positron and the electron took place. Recordings are simultaneously made along several planes, and the intersections of these planes identify the location of the source of the radiation. Because the camera records the location of the collision rather than the location of the initial release of the positron, the capacity to pinpoint the exact location in which the chemical is being used is somewhat limited.

There are several positive characteristics of PET imaging that contribute to its usefulness. Spatial resolution ranges from 1–2 mm. Time needed to obtain adequate PET data regarding different aspects of neural functioning ranges from 70 seconds for cerebral blood flow studies to over 40 minutes for studies of intracellular and neurotransmitter activities. PET images can reflect various activities within the brain, depending on what type of radioactive isotopes are used. Blood flow, oxygen use, glucose metabolism, and specific neurotransmitters can all be studied using PET imaging. In addition, PET can identify the activity of intracellular activities associated with neuronal action (Kessler, 2003). Some PET measures are more directly connected to glucose and oxygen consumption than are fMRI measures, which rely on the correlation between blood flow and the other neuronal processes; PET imaging is therefore more reliable when there are questions regarding ties between blood flow and other processes. For example, PET research has demonstrated that oxygen metabolism and blood flow are poorly correlated during some visualization tasks, apparently because glucose is sometimes metabolized without oxygenation (Huettel et al., 2004).

Despite its strengths as an imaging tool, PET also has important weaknesses that limit its use. Because PET assesses the location at which the gamma photons are generated rather than the point at which the isotope is used, the spatial resolution for PET images is poorer than for fMRI. Because PET images require the use of radioactive isotopes, the number of times a subject can safely pass through the procedure is limited. PET images require the on-site availability of a cyclotron where the isotopes can be created, which limits the number of locations where PET can be used. Finally, many photon emissions are needed in order to create a PET image, so the range of time needed to collect output in a single session can range from 90 seconds to 40 minutes and more, depending on the rate of decay of the isotope; temporal specificity of PET is therefore limited (Huettel *et al.*, 2004; Posner & Raichle, 1994).

Single photon emission computed tomography (SPECT)

Single photon emission computed tomography is similar to PET in many ways, although there are basic differences in the process whereby the image of functioning is created. SPECT involves the measurement of radiation resulting from decay of radioactive isotopes introduced into the brain. Different isotopes are associated with different neural processes, and they therefore offer indications of different aspects of neural function. SPECT differs from PET in that SPECT radiation results from SPECT isotopes "capturing" electrons at the site where the isotope is located, and subsequently releasing a single photon from that site; the released photon can then be measured using a SPECT camera. While PET cameras record all radiation events involving two photons moving in opposite directions, SPECT cameras record single photons moving in one direction along identifiable parallel planes, rejecting photons that are not moving in the identified plane (see Dougherty *et al.*, 2004, pp. 76–7). PET and SPECT technologies both then identify individual voxels in three dimensions based on recording radiation moving along various specified planes. Because PET records all radiation, and SPECT involves rejection of radiation not moving along identified planes, SPECT spatial resolution falls between 5–6 mm, which is significantly lower than images offered by PET or fMRI (Kessler, 2003).

SPECT is used to examine blood flow and various aspects of neurotransmitter activity. SPECT is not used to examine glucose metabolism. SPECT frequently requires a longer time for collection of data, and as a result is limited with regard to obtaining repeated measurements of neuronal activity in a single setting. SPECT is therefore not typically used to assess regional blood flow during specific tasks because often only one image can be collected per day. With PET and fMRI, multiple images can be collected over the course of a day, allowing for repeated assessment of brain activity. At times the choice to use SPECT rather than PET is based on the more widespread availability of SPECT machinery.

Functional magnetic resonance imaging (fMRI)

Functional magnetic resonance imaging applies the MRI technology to changes in blood flow associated with brain activity. Basic MRI technology applies also to fMRI. fMRI is based on the fact that blood saturated with oxygen has lower magnetic susceptibility than blood that has been depleted of oxygen. The BOLD (blood-oxygenation-level-dependent) fMRI is based on the observation that activation of an area of the brain leads to a predictable pattern of changes in levels of oxygen saturation in blood flowing through the area. These changes lead to changes in the MRI signal that are associated with brain activity. fMRI images do not directly reflect depletion of blood oxygen due to oxygen consumption during activity in neurons. Instead, neuronal activity triggers complex changes in constriction of blood vessels and in rate of blood flow. It is these changes in blood flow that are reflected in fMRI images. While it is clear that neural activity affects regional blood flow, and that fMRI images are correlated with neural activity, the nature of the relationships between neural activity, blood flow, and fMRI images remains the focus of debate and research (Heuttel *et al.*, 2004; Kessler, 2003).

Positive characteristics of fMRI have resulted in its rapidly increasing use as a tool for imaging brain activity. Spatial resolution can range from 1–3 mm. Temporal resolution currently stands at about 6 seconds. There is no known radiation hazard, so multiple scanning repetitions can be initiated during a single assessment session as well as over the long term.

Despite its strengths, there are limitations to the usefulness of fMRI. Because it is based on flood flow, it is somewhat removed from the actual activity of interest within and between neurons. It is not an effective way to measure glucose metabolism, and it does not offer ways to assess activity at specific locations within and between neurons. There are indications that important neural processes during cognitive activities do not rely on oxygen, especially during early steps of processing, and measures of blood flow may therefore not help explain these activities (Huettel *et al.*, 2004). While the speed of fMRI is much faster than that of PET or SPECT, changes that occur during cognitive processing occur at the rate of tens of milliseconds rather than 5 or 6 seconds, so fMRI temporal sensitivity does not allow analysis of such rapid activity.

In the relatively few years it has been used in assessment, fMRI has been used to examine a wide variety of aspects of brain function. It has been used to assess development of the visual system, language production, and various executive functions, including impulse control, working memory, and problem solving (Kessler, 2003). Experiments using fMRI have been carried out to examine activation of the hippocampus while using various episodic memory retrieval strategies (Huettel *et al.*, 2004). fMRI techniques appear particularly useful in mapping the interactions of various areas of the brain while completing specific types of complex tasks.

Other imaging techniques

The imaging techniques reviewed in this Appendix are the ones most frequently used in research as well as clinical work. Other techniques are available, but are not so widely used. These will not be explored here. Two examples are magnetic resonance spectroscopy (MRS) and magnetoencephalography (MEG) (Huettel *et al.*, 2004; Kessler, 2003). In addition, there are multiple specific modifications of the techniques described in this Appendix that are based on alterations in technology or data analysis, and these specific modifications support unique strategies. It can also be expected that new neuroimaging strategies will be identified and applied rapidly in the future.

Strategies in neuroimaging research

Traditional research strategies, for example, comparing images obtained from impaired subjects with images obtained from normal subjects, are used in reseach based on neuroimaging. However, there are two strategies in conducting neuroscience research using neuroimaging techniques that should be mentioned in order to complete this review. The first is the strategy of paired image subtraction (Posner & Raichle, 1994). The second is the strategy of converging operations (Huettel *et al.*, 2004). While neither of these operations is necessarily limited to studies involving neuroimaging, their widespread use and importance in neuroscience research makes it important to discuss them.

Paired image subtraction involves collecting data from subjects at rest and then subtracting that data from data obtained from subjects while they complete a specific task. For example, a subject could be asked to watch a stationary visual stimulus, and then be asked to watch the same stimulus in motion (Posner & Raichle, 1994). Blood flow measurements obtained during the first task could then be subtracted from blood flow measurements taken during the second task. The result is assumed to indicate what parts of the brain become active solely because of the introduction of motion. Studies involving all types of neuroimaging techniques rely on this strategy to determine the contribution of particular areas of the brain to specific tasks.

Converging operations refers to the use of multiple types of neuroimaging techniques to examine a single process, with the strengths of each type of technique being used to identify specific details of the process. Posner and Raichle (1994) offered a clear explanation using this approach to integrate PET imaging with EEG recordings to help identify the series of locations in the brain used to process either visual–spatial characteristics of typed words, or the meaning associated with the same typed words. The specificity of location offered by PET images was combined with the temporal specificity offered by EEG technology to yield a much clearer identification of the locations of action and speed of neural processing that accompany visual–spatial analysis as compared to analysis of meaning. Since the time that Posner and Raichle wrote their explanation, new technologies have been added to research techniques being used, and complex computer programs have been developed that allow integration of spatially explicit MRI data with PET or fMRI data that offer specific identification of function over time (Huettel et al., 2004). This integration of technology supports the mapping of fMRI data onto MRI images of the same brain, and subsequently correlating this integration with a standard atlas of brain structure that facilitates comparisons between subjects.

Conclusion

Integration of data gathered using different neuroimaging techniques will continue to enrich the understanding of the brain. Specifically relevant to the current application of neuroscience to understanding psychological therapies, neuroimaging is likely to contribute rapidly to understanding of particular processes involved in psychotherapy (Roffman et al., 2005). Neuroimaging is likely to guide more complete elaboration of the ideas regarding psychotherapy presented in this book, and it also likely to contribute to significantly altering some of the ideas proposed herein. It is likely to provide new process and outcome measures for psychotherapy, and it is likely to lead to development of more effective psychotherapy techniques (Fonagy, 2004). Maintaining an understanding of neuroimaging techniques will help clinicians apply new developments to clinical practice more rapidly and more effectively.

References

Alexander, F. & French, T. M. (1946). *Psychoanalytic Therapy*. New York: Ronald Press Co.

Amen, D. G. (2004). *Images of human behavior: A brain SPECT atlas*. Newport Beach, California: Mindworks Press.

Andersen, S. L. & Teicher, M. H. (2004). Delayed effects of early stress on hippocampal development. *Neuropsychopharmocology*, **29**, 1988–1993.

Arciero, G. & Guidano, V. F. (2000). Experience, explanation, and the quest for coherence. In R. A. Neimeyer & R. D. Raskin, eds., *Constructions of Disorder: Meaning-making Frameworks for Psychotherapy*. Washington, DC: American Psychological Association.

Arnold, S. E. (1999). Neurodevelopmental abnormalities in schizophrenia: insights from neuropathology. *Development and Psychopathology*, **11**, 439–56.

Bandura, A. (1977). *Social Learning Theory*. Englewood Cliffs, NJ: Prentice-Hall.

Barlow, D. H. (1988). *Anxiety and Its Disorders: The Nature and Treatment of Anxiety and Panic*. New York: The Guilford Press.

Basbaum, A. I. & Jessell, T. M. (2000). The perception of pain. In E. R. Kandel, J. H. Schwartz & T. M. Jessel, eds., *Priciples of Neural Science*, 4th edn. Norwalk, CT: Appleton & Lange, pp. 472–91.

Bauer, P. J. (2004). Getting explicit memory off the ground: steps toward construction of a neuro-developmental account of changes in the first two years of life. *Developmental Review*, **24**, 347–73.

Beck, A. T. (1976). *Cognitive Therapy and the Emotional Disorders*. New York: International Universities Press.

Bellack, A. S. (2004). Skills training for people with severe mental illness. *Psychiatric Rehabilitation Journal*, **27**(4), 375–91.

Bellack, A. S., Hersen, M. & Kazdin, A. E. (eds.) (1990). *International Handbook of Behavior Modification and Therapy*. New York: Plenum.

Bennett, E. L., Diamond, M. C., Krech, D. & Rosenzweig, M. R. (1964). Chemical and anatomical plasticity of brain. *Science*, **146**, 610–19.

Berka, C., Levendowski, D. J., Cvetinovic, M. M., *et al.* (2004). Real-time analysis of EEG indexes of alertness, cognition, and memory acquired with a wireless EEG headset. *International Journal of Human–Computer Interaction*, **17**(2), 151–70.

Blanchard, R. J., Yudko, E. B., Rodgers, R. J. & Blanchard, C. D. (1993). Defense system psychopharmocology: an ethological approach to the pharmacology of fear and anxiety. *Behavioural Brain Research*, **58**, 155–65.

Boersma, K., den Hengst, S., Dekker, J. & Emmelkamp, P. (1976). Exposure and response prevention in the natural environment: a comparison with obsessive–compulsive patients. *Behaviour Research and Therapy*, **14**, 19–24.

Borkovec, T. D., Wilkinson, L., Folensbee, R. & Lerman, C. (1983). Stimulus control applications to the treatment of worry. *Behaviour Research and Therapy*, **21**(3), 247–51.

Bowers, D., Bauer, R. M. & Heilman, K. M. (1993). The nonverbal affect lexicon: theoretical perspectives from neuropsychological studies of affect perception. *Neuropsychology*, **17**(4), 433–44.

Bowlby, J. (1973). *Attachment and loss (Volume II). Separation: anxiety and anger.* New York: Basic Books.

Bremner, J. D., Southwick, S. M., Johnson, D. R., Yehuda, R. & Charney, D. S. (1993). Childhood physical abuse and combat-related posttraumatic stress disorder in Vietnam veterans. *American Journal of Psychiatry*, **150**, 235–39.

Breslau, N., Chilcoat, H. D., Kessler, R. C. & Davis, G. C. (1999). Previous exposure to trauma and PTSD effects of subsequent trauma: results from the Detroit area survey of trauma. *American Journal of Psychiatry*, **156**(6), 902–07.

Carter, W. R., Johnson, M. C. & Borkovec, T. D. (1986). Worry: An electrocortical analysis. *Advances in Behavioural Research and Therapy*, **8**, 193–204.

Casey, B. J., Giedd, J. N. & Thomas, K. M. (2000). Structural and functional brain development and its relation to cognitive development. *Biological Psychology*, **54**, 241–57.

Caspi, A., Sugden, K., Moffitt, T. E., *et al.* (2003). Influence of life stress on depression: moderation by a polymorphism in the 5-HTT gene. *Science*, **301**, 386–389.

Chklovskii, D. B., Mel, B. W. & Svoboda, K. (2004). Cortical rewiring and information storage. *Nature*, **431**, 782–88.

Christensen, B. K., Carney, C. E. & Segal, Z. V. (2006). Cognitive processing models of depression. In D. J. Stein, D. J. Kupfer & A. F. Schatzberg, eds., *Textbook of Mood Disorders*. Washington, DC: American Psychiatric Publishing, Inc., pp. 131–44.

Chugani, H. T. & Chugani, D. C. (1997). Positron emission tomography studies of developing brain. In M. S. Keshavan & R. M. Murray, eds., *Neurodevelopment and Adult Psychopathology*. Cambridge: Cambridge University Press, pp. 93–103.

Cicchetti, D. & Cannon, T. D. (1999). Neurodevelopmental processes in the ontogenesis and epigenesis of psychopathology. *Development and Psychopathology*, **11**, 375–93.

Coulson, S. & Van Petten, C. (2002). Conceptual integration and metaphor: an event-related potential study. *Memory and Cognition*, **30**(6), 958–68.

Cozolino, L. (2002). *The Neuroscience of Psychotherapy: Building and Rebuilding the Human Brain*. New York: W. W. Norton & Company.

Dawson, G., Frey, K., Self, J., *et al.* (1999). Frontal brain electrical activity in infants of depressed and nondepressed mothers: relation to variations in infant behavior. *Development and Psychopathology*, **11**, 589–605.

De Bellis, M. D. (2001). Developmental traumatology: the psychobiological development of maltreated children and its implications for research, treatment, and policy. *Development and Psychopathology*, **13**, 539–64.

Deffenbacher, J. L., Oetting, E. R. & DiGiuseppe, R. A. (2002). Principles of empirically supported interventions applied to anger management. *Counseling Psychologist*, **30**(2), 262–80.

Derryberry, C. & Tucker, D. M. (1992). Neural mechanisms of emotion. *Journal of Consulting and Clinical Psychology*, **60**(3), 329–38.

Desantis, A., Coster, W., Bigsby, R. & Lester, B. (2004). Colic and fussing in infancy, and sensory processing at 3 to 8 years of age. *Infant Mental Health Journal*, **25**(6), 522–39.

Dobson, K. S. (2003). *Handbook of Cognitive–Behavioral Therapies*, 2nd edn. New York: The Guilford Press.

Dolan, R. J. (2000). Functional neuroimaging of the human amygdala during emotional processing and learning. In J. P. Aggleton, ed., *The Amygdala: A Functional Analysis*, 2nd edn. Oxford: Oxford University Press, pp. 631–53.

Dolcos, F., Graham, R., Labar, K. & Cabeza, R. (2003). Coactivation of the amygdala and hippocampus predicts better recall for emotional than for neutral pictures. *Brain and Cognition*, **51**, 221–23.

Dougherty, D. D., Rauch, S. L. & Fischman, A. J. (2004). Positron emission tomography and single photon emission computed tomography. In D. D. Dougherty, S. L. Rauch & J. F. Rosenbaum, eds., *Essentials of neuroimaging for clinical practice*. Washington DC: American Psychiatric Publishing, Inc, pp. 75–91.

Durston, S., Pol, H. E. H., Casey, B. J., Giedd, J. N., Buitelaar, J. K. & van Engeland, H. (2001). Anatomical MRI of the developing human brain: What have we learned? *Journal of the American Academy of Child and Adolescent Psychiatry*, **40**(9), 1012–20.

Farah, M. J. (1989). The neural basis of mental imagery. *Trends in Neuroscience*, **12**(10), 395–99.

Fenichel, O. (1945). *The Psychoanalytic Theory of Neurosis*. New York: W. W. Norton & Company.

Foa, E. B. & Chambless, D. L. (1978). Habituation of subjective anxiety during flooding in imagery. *Behaviour Research and Therapy*, **16**, 391–99.

Foa, E. B., Rothbaum, B. O., Riggs, D. S. & Murdock, T. B. (1991). Treatment of posttraumatic stress disorder in rape victims: a comparison between cognitive behavioral procedures and counseling. *Journal of Consulting and Clinical Psychology*, **59**, 715–23.

Foa, E. B., Steketee, B. S., Grayson, J. B., Turner, R. M. & Latimer, P. R. (1984). Deliberate exposure and blocking of obsessive-compulsive rituals: immediate and long term effects. *Behavior Therapy*, **15**, 450–72.

Fonagy, P. (2004). Psychotherapy meets neuroscience. *Psychiatric Bulletin*, **28**, 357–59.

Ford, J. D. (2005). Treatment implications of altered affect regulation and information processing following child maltreatment. *Psychiatric Annals*, **35**(5), 410–19.

Freedman, D. A. (1981). The effect of sensory and other deficits in children on their experience of people. *Journal of the American Psychoanalytic Society*, **29**, 831–67.

Gabbard, G. O. (2004). *Long-term Psychodynamic Psychotherapy: A Basic Text*. Washington, DC: American Psychiatric Publishing, Inc.

Gilliam, T. C., Kandel, E. R. & Jessell, T. M. (2000). Genes and Behavior. In E. R Kandel, J. H. Schwartz & T. M. Jessell, eds., *Principles of Neural Science*, 4th edn. Norwalk, CT: Appleton & Lange, pp. 36–62.

Glaser, D. (2000). Child abuse and neglect and the brain—a review. *Journal of Child Psychology and Psychiatry*, **41**(1), 97–116.

Goldstein, M. A. & Price, B. H. (2004). Magnetic resonance imaging. In D. D Dougherty, S. L. Rauch & J. F. Rosenbaum, eds., *Essentials of Neuroimaging for Clinical Practice*. Washington, DC: American Psychiatric Publishing, Inc, pp. 21–73.

Graf, P., Squire, L. R. & Mandler, G. (1984). The information that amnesic patients do not forget. *Journal of Experimental Psychology: Learning, Memory, & Cognition*, **10**(1), 164–78.

Gray, J. A. (1982). *The Neuropsychology of Anxiety: An Enquiry into the Functions of the Septo-hippocampal System*. New York: Oxford University Press.

Gray, J. A. & McNaughton, N. (2003). *The Neuropsychology of Anxiety: An Enquiry into the Functions of the Septo-hippocampal System*, 2nd edn. Oxford: Oxford University Press.

Greenberg, L. S. (1980). The intensive analysis of recurring events from the practice of Gestalt therapy. *Psychotherapy: Theory, Research and Practice*, **17**(2), 143–52.

Greenough, W. T. & Black, J. E. (1992). Induction of brain structure by experience: Substrates for cognitive development. In M. R. Gunnar & C. A. Nelson, eds., *Developmental Behavioral Science: The Minnesota Symposia on Child Psychology (Vol. 24)*. Hillsdale, New Jersey: Lawrence Erlbaum Associates, Publishers, pp. 155–200.

Greenough, W. T., Black, J. E. & Wallace, C. S. (1987). Experience and brain development. *Child Development*, **58**(3), 539–59.

Guerri, C. (1998). Neuroanatomical and neurophysiological mechanisms involved in central nervous system dysfunctions induced by prenatal alcohol exposure. *Alcoholism: Clinical and Experimental Research*, **22**(2), 304–12.

Guidano, V. F. & Liotti, G. (1983). *Cognitive Processes and Emotional Disorders*. New York: Guilford Press.

Hasler, D., Drevets, W. C., Manji, H. K. & Charney, D. S. (2004). Discovering endophenotypes for major depression. *Neuropsychopharmacology*, **29**, 1765–81.

Hayashi, A., Nagaoka, M., Yamada, K., Ichitani, Y., Miake, Y. & Okado, M. (1998). Maternal stress induces synaptic loss and developmental disabilities of offspring. *International Journal of Neuroscience*, **16**(3/4), 209–16.

Heilman, K. M. & Valenstein, E. (eds.) (1985). *Clinical Neuropsychology*, 2nd edn. New York: Oxford University Press.

Howieson, D. B., Loring, D. W. & Hannay, H. J. (2004). Neurobehavioral variables and diagnostic issues. In M. D. Lezak, D. B. Howieson & D. W. Loring, eds., *Neuropsychological Assessment*, 4th edn. New York: Oxford University Press, pp. 286–336.

Hubel, D. H. & Wiesel, T. N. (1959). Receptive fields of single neurons in the cat's striate cortex. *Journal of Physiology*, **148**, 574–91.

Hubel, D. H. & Wiesel, T. N. (1970). The period of susceptibility to the physiological effects of unilateral eye closure in kittens. *Journal of Physiology*, **206**, 419–36.

Huettel, S. A., Song, A. W. & McCarthy, G. (2004). *Functional Magnetic Resonance Imaging*. Sunderland, MA: Sinaure Associates, Inc.

Jacobs, W. J. & Nadel, L. (1998). Neurobiology of reconstructed memory. *Psychology, Public Policy, and Law*, **4**(4), 1110–34.

Jacobson, S. W. (1998). Specificity of neurobehavioral outcomes associated with prenatal alcohol exposure. *Alcoholism: Clinical and Experimental Research*, **22**(2), 313–20.

Janicak, P. G., Davis, J. M., Preskorn, S. H. & Ayd, F. J. (2001). *Principles and Practice of Psychopharmacology*, 3rd edn. Philadelphia, PA: Lippincott Williams & Wilkins.

Johnston, M. V. (2004). Clinical disorders of brain plasticity. *Brain and Development*, **26**, 73–80.

Kandel, E. R. (1998). A new intellectual framework for psychiatry. *American Journal of Psychiatry*, **155**(4), 457–69.

Kandel, E. R. (2000). Cellular mechanisms of learning and the biological basis of individuality. In E. R. Kandel, J. H. Schwartz & T. M. Jessell, eds., *Principles of Neural Science*, 4th edn. Norwalk, CT: Appleton & Lange, pp. 1247–79.

Kandel, E. R., Kupfermann, I. & Iversen, S. (2000a). Learning and memory. In E. R. Kandel, J. H. Schwartz & T. M. Jessell, eds., *Principles of Neural Science*, 4th edn. Norwalk, CT: Appleton & Lange, pp. 1227–46.

Kandel, E. R., Schwartz, J. H. & Jessell, T. M. (eds.) (2000b). *Principles of Neural Science*, 4th edn. Norwalk, CT: Appleton & Lange.

Kendell, R. E. (1999). Much diversity, many categories, no entities. In M. Maj & N. Sartorius, eds., *Depressive Disorders*. Chichester: John Wiley & Sons, pp. 52–4.

Kessler, R. M. (2003). Imaging methods for evaluating brain function in man. *Neurobiology of Aging*, **24**(Supplement 1), S21–S35.

Kinniburgh, K. J., Blaustein, M. & Spinazzola, J. (2005). Attachment, self-regulation, and competency. *Psychiatric Annals*, **35**(5), 424–30.

Klein, D. N., Shankman, S. A. & McFarland, B. F. (2006). Classification of mood disorders. In D. J. Stein, D. J. Kupfer & A. F. Schatzberg, eds., *Textbook of Mood Disorder*. Washington, DC: American Psychiatric Publishing, Inc, pp. 17–32.

Knudsen, E. I. (2004). Sensitive periods in the development of the brain and behavior, *Journal of Cognitive Neuroscience*, **16**(8): 1412–25.

Kofman, O. (2002). The role of prenatal stress in the etiology of developmental behavioural disorders. *Neuroscience and Biobehavioural Reviews*, **26**, 457–70.

Kotrla, K. J., Sater, A. K. & Weinberger, D. R. (1997). Neuropathology, neurodevelopment, and schizophrenia. In M. S. Keshavan & R. M. Murray, eds., *Neurodevelopment and Adult Psychopathology*. Cambridge: Cambridge University Press, pp. 187–98.

Kramer, D. A. (2005). Commentary: gene–environment interplay in the context of genetics, epigenetics, and gene expression. *Journal of the American Academy of Child and Adolescent Psychiatry*, **44**(10), 19–27.

Krasner, L. (1990). History of behavior modification. In A. S. Bellack, M. Hersen & A. E. Kazdin, eds., *International Handbook of Behavior Modification and Therapy*, 2nd edn. New York: Plenum Press, pp. 3–25.

Kuperberg, G. R. (2004). Electroencephalography, event-related potentials, and magnetoencephalography. In D. D. Dougherty, S. L. Rauch & J. F. Rosenbaum, eds., *Essentials of Neuroimaging for Clinical Practice*. Washington, DC: American Psychiatric Publishing, Inc, pp. 117–27.

Lambert, M. J. (2004). *Bergin and Garfield's Handbook of Psychotherapy and Behavior Change*. New York: John Wiley & Sons, Inc.

Lang, P. J. (1979). A bioinformational theory of emotional imagery. *Psychophysiology*, **16**, 495–512.

Lanius, R. A., Williamson, P. C., Densmore, M., *et al.* (2004). The nature of traumatic memories: a 4-T fMRI functional connectivity analysis. *American Journal of Psychiatry*, **161**, 36–44.

LeDoux, J. (1996). *The Emotional Brain: The Mysterious Underpinnings of Emotional Life*. New York: Simon & Schuster.

LeDoux, J. (2002). *Synaptic Self: How Our Brains Become Who We Are*. New York: Penguin Putnam Inc.

Levin, H. S. (2003). Neuroplasticity following non-penetrating traumatic brain injury. *Brain Injury*, **17**(8), 665–74.

Levine, D. S. (2000). *Introduction to Neural and Cognitive Modeling*, 2nd edn. Mahwah, NJ: Lawrence Erlbaum Associates, Publishers.

Lezak, M. D., Howieson, D. B. & Loring, D. W. (2004). *Neuropsychological Assessment*, 4th edn. New York: Oxford University Press.

Loftus, E. F. (2005). Searching for the neurobiology of the misinformation effect. *Learning & Memory*, **12**, 1–2.

Loftus, E. F. & Hoffman, H. G. (1989). Misinformation and memory: the creation of new memories. *Journal of Experimental Psychology: General*, **118**(1), 100–4.

Luria, A. (1966). *Higher Cortical Functions in Man*. New York: Basic Books.

MacLean, P. D. (1990). *The Triune Brain in Evolution: Role in Paleocerebral Functions*. New York: Plenum Press.

Mahler, M. S., Pine, F. & Bergman, A. (1975). *The Psychological Birth of the Human Infant: Separation and Individuation*. New York: Basic Books, Inc.

Mahoney, M. J. (1974). *Cognition and Behavior Modification*. Cambridge, MA: Ballinger Publishing Company.

Maj, M. & Sartorius, N. (eds.) (1999). *Depressive Disorders*. Chichester: John Wiley & Sons, Ltd.

Marin, O. & Rubenstein, J. L. R. (2003). Cell migration in the forebrain. *Annual Review of Neuroscience*, **26**, 441–83.

Mayberg, H. S., Keightley, M., Mahurin, R. K. & Brannan, S. K. (2002). Neuropsychiatric aspects of mood and affective disorders. In S. C. Yudofsky & R. E. Hales, eds., *Neuropsychiatry and Clinical Neurosciences*. Washington, DC: American Psychiatric Publishing, Inc, pp. 1021–48.

McGaugh, J. L. (2004). The amygdala modulates the consolidation of memories of emotionally arousing experiences. *Annual Review of Neuroscience*, **27**, 1–28.

McNaughton, N. & Corr, P.J. (2004). A two-dimensional neuropsychology of defense: fear/anxiety and defensive distance. *Neuroscience and Biobehavioral Reviews*, **28**, 285–305.

Mersch, P.P.A., Emmelkamp, P.M.G. & Lips, C. (1991). Social phobia: individual response patterns and the long-term effects of behavioral and cognitive interventions. A follow-up study. *Behaviour Research and Therapy*, **29**(4), 357–62.

Mitchell, B.D., Emsley, J.G., Magavi, S.S.P., Arlotta, P. & Macklis, J.D. (2004). Constitutive and induced neurogenesis in the adult mammalian brain: manipulation of endogenous precursors toward CNS repair. *Developmental Neuroscience*, **26**(2–4), 101–17.

Monroe, S.M. & Harkness, K.L. (2005). Life stress, the "kindling" hypothesis, and the recurrence of depression: Considerations from a life stress perspective, *Psychological Review*, **112**(2): 417–45.

Nagy, Z., Westerberg, H. & Klingberg, T. (2004). Maturation of white matter is associated with the development of cognitive functions during childhood. *Journal of Cognitive Neuroscience*, **16**(7), 1227–33.

Newport, E.L. (1990). Maturational constraints on language learning. *Cognitive Science*, **14**(1), 11–28.

O'Connor, T.G., Marvin, R.S., Rutter, M., Olrick, J.T., Britner, P.A. & the English and Romanian adoptees study team (2003). Child–parent attachment following early institutional deprivation. *Development and Psychopathology*, **15**, 19–38.

Okado, Y. & Stark, C.E.L. (2005). Neural activity during encoding predicts false memories created by misinformation. *Learning & Memory*, **12**, 3–11.

O'Keefe, J. & Nadel, L. (1978). *The Hippocampus as a Cognitive Map*. Oxford: Clarendon Press.

O'Keefe, J. & Nadel, L. (1979). Precis of O'Keefe & Nadel's *The Hippocampus as Cognitive Map*. *The Behavioral and Brain Sciences*, **2**, 487–533.

Paolino, T.F. (1981). *Psychoanalytic Psychotherapy: Theory, Technique, Therapeutic Relationship and Treatability*. New York: Brunner/Mazel.

Paris, J. (2005). Understanding self-mutilation in borderline personality disorder. *Harvard Review of Psychiatry*, **13**(3), 179–85.

Park, L.T. & Gonzalez, R.G. (2004). Computed tomography. In D.D. Dougherty, S.L. Rauch & J.F. Rosenbaum, eds., *Essentials of Neuroimaging for Clinical Practice*. Washington, DC: American Psychiatric Publishing, Inc, pp. 1–19.

Physicians' Desk Reference, 57th edn. (2003). Montvale, NJ: Thomson PDR.

Pliszka, S.R. (2003). *Neuroscience for the Mental Health Clinician*. New York: The Guilford Press.

Plomin, R. & McGuffin, P. (2003). Psychopathology in the postgenomic era. *Annual Review of Psychology*, **54**, 205–28.

Posner, M.I. & Raichle, M.E. (1994). *Images of Mind*. New York: Scientific American Library.

Post, R.M. (1992). Transduction of psychosocial stress into the neurobiology of recurrent affective disorder. *American Journal of Psychiatry*, **149**, 999–1010.

Purves, D. & Lichtman, J.W. (1985). *Principles of Neural Development*. Sunderland, MA: Sinauer Associates, Inc.

Rakos, R. F. (1991). *Assertive Behavior: Theory, Research, and Training*. London: Routledge.

Reik, T. (1948). *Listening With The Third Ear: The Inner Experience of a Psychoanalyst*. New York: Farrar, Straus & Company.

Reuter-Lorenz, P. A. (2002). New visions of the aging mind and brain. *Trends in Cognitive Neuroscience*, **6**(9), 394–400.

Roffman, J. L., Marci, C. D., Glick, D. M., Dougherty, D. D. & Rauch, S. L. (2005). Neuroimaging and the functional neuroanatomy of psychotherapy. *Psychological Medicine*, **35**, 1–14.

Roozendaal, B. (2002). Stress and memory: opposing effects of glucocorticoids on memory consolidation and memory retrieval. *Neurobiology of Learning and Memory*, **78**, 578–595.

Rutter, M. (2005). Environmentally mediated risks for psychopathology: research strategies and findings. *Journal of the Academy of Child and Adolescent Psychiatry*, **44**(1), 3–18.

Saper, C. B. (2000). Brain stem modulation of sensation, movement, and consciousness. In E. R. Kandel, J. H. Schwartz & T. M. Jessell, eds., *Principles of Neural Science*, 4th edn. Norwalk, CT: Appleton & Lange, pp. 889–909.

Saper, C. B., Iversen, S. & Frackowiak, R. (2000). Integration of sensory and motor function: the association areas of the cerebral cortex and the cognitive capabilities of the brain. In E. R. Kandel, J. H. Schwartz & T. M. Jessell, eds., *Principles of Neural Science*, 4th edn. Norwalk, CT: Appleton & Lange, pp. 349–80.

Scahill, L. & Martin, A. (2001). Pediatric psychopharmacology II: General principles, specific drug treatments, and clinical practice. In M. Lewis, ed., *Child and Adolescent Psychiatry: A Comprehensive Textbook*, 3rd edn. Philadelphia, Pennsylvania: Lippincott, Williams & Wilkins, pp. 951–74.

Schacter, D. L. & Tulving, E. (eds.) (1994). *Memory Systems 1994*. Cambridge, MA: The MIT Press.

Schmidt-Hieber, C., Jonas, P. & Bischofberger, J. (2004). Enhanced synaptic plasticity in newly generated granule cells of the adult hippocampus. *Nature*, **429**(6988), 143–87.

Schore, A. N. (1994). *Affect Regulation and the Origin of the Self: The Neurobiology of Emotional Development*. Hillsdale, NJ: Laurence Erlbaum Associates.

Schwartz, J. H., & Westbrook, G. L. (2000). The cytology of neurons. In E. R. Kandel, J. H. Schwartz & T. M. Jessell, eds., *Principles of Neural Science*, 4th edn. Norwalk, CT: Appleton & Lange, pp. 67–87.

Seitz, A. R. & Watanabe, T. (2003). Is subliminal learning really passive? *Nature*, **422**(6927), 36.

Shalak, L. & Perlman, J. M. (2004). Hypoxic—ischemic brain injury in the term infant – current concepts. *Early Human Development*, **80**, 125–41.

Shapiro, F. (1995). *Eye Movement Desensitization and Reprocessing*. New York: The Guilford Press.

Siegel, D. J. (1999). *The Developing Mind: How Relationships and the Brain Interact to Shape Who We Are*. New York: The Guilford Press.

Smith, E. W. L. (1976). *The Growing Edge of Gestalt Therapy*. New York: Brunner/Mazel.

Squire, L. F. (1992). Memory and the hippocampus: a synthesis from findings with rats, monkeys, and humans. *Psychological Review*, **99**(2), 195–231.

Squire, L. F., Knowlton, B. & Musen, G. (1993). The structure and organization of memory. *Annual Review of Psychology*, **44**, 453–95.

Southwick, S. M., Vythilingam, M. & Charney, D. S. (2005). The psychobiology of depression and resilience to stress: implications for prevention and treatment. *Annual Review of Clinical Psychology*, **1**, 255–91.

Stahl, S. M. (2000). *Essential Psychopharmacology: Neuroscientific Basis and Practical Applications*. Cambridge: Cambridge University Press.

Stein, D. J., Kupfer, D. J. & Schatzberg, A. F. (eds.) (2006). *Textbook of Mood Disorders*. Washington, DC: American Psychiatric Publishing, Inc.

Stern, D. A. (1985). *The Interpersonal World of the Infant: A View from Psychoanalysis and Developmental Psychology*. New York: Basic Book, Inc.

Teicher, M. H., Dumont, N. L., Ito, Y., Vaituzis, C., Giedd, J. N. & Andersen, S. L. (2004). Childhood neglect is associated with reduced corpus callosum area. *Biological Psychiatry*, **56**, 80–5.

Teeter, P. A. & Semrud-Clikeman, M. (1997). *Child neuropsychology: assessment and interventions for neurodevelopmental disorders*. Boston: Allyn and Bacon.

Tsien, J. Z., Huerta, P. T. & Tonegawa, S. (1996). The essential role of hippocampal CA1 NMDA receptor-dependent synaptic plasticity in spatial memory. *Cell*, **87**, 1327–38.

Vaughan, S. C. (1997). *The Talking Cure: Why Traditional Talking Therapy Offers a Better Chance for Long-term Relief Than Any Drug*. New York: Henry Holt and Company.

Watson, C. (1995). *Basic Human Neuroanatomy: An introductory atlas (5th edition)*, Boston, MA: Little, Brown and Company.

Watson, J. B., Mednick, S. A., Huttunen, M. & Wang, X. (1999). Prenatal teratogens and the development of adult mental illness. *Development and Psychopathology*, **11**, 457–66.

Weinberger, N. M. (2004). Specific long-term memory traces in primary auditory cortex. *Nature Reviews Neuroscience*, **5**(4), 279–90.

Westbrook, G. L. (2000). Seizures and epilepsy. In E. R. Kandel, J. H. Schwartz & T. M. Jessell, eds., *Principles of Neural Science*, 4th edn. Norwalk, CT: Appleton & Lange, pp. 910–35.

Wiltgen, B. J., Brown, R. A. M., Talton, L. E. & Silva, A. J. (2004). New circuits for old memories: the role of the neocortex in consolidation. *Neuron*, **44**, 101–8.

Wolpe, J. (1958). *Psychotherapy by Reciprocal Inhibition*. Stanford, CA: Stanford University Press.

Yakolev, P. I. & Lecours, A. R. (1967). Morphological criteria of growth and maturation of the nervous system in man. In A. Minkowski, ed., *Regional Development of the Brain in Early Life*. Oxford: Blackwell Scientific Publications, pp. 3–65.

Yerkes, R. M. & Dodson, J. D. (1908). The relation of strength of stimulus to rapidity of habit-formation. *Journal of Comparative Neurology and Psychology*, **18**, 459–82.

Zajonc, R. C. (1980). Feeling and thinking: preferences need no inferences. *American Psychologist*, **35**(2), 151–75.

Zubicaray, G. I., McMahon, K. & Wilson, S. J. (2001). Brain activity during the encoding, retention, and retrieval of stimulus representations. *Learning and Memory*, **8**(5), 243–51.

Index